Nutrition

A SCOPE® PUBLICATION

Mohamed el Lozy, MD
Assistant Professor of Nutrition
Department of Nutrition
School of Public Health
Harvard University

M. Guillermo Herrera, MD
Associate Professor of Medicine
Department of Nutrition
School of Public Health
Harvard University

Michael C. Latham, MD
Professor of International Nutrition
Cornell University

Robert B. McGandy, MD
Professor of Nutrition
Clinical Professor of Pathology
Tufts University

Mary B. McCann, MD
Resident in Psychiatry
Maine Medical Center
Portland

Fredrick J. Stare, MD
Professor of Nutrition
Founder and Former Chairman
Department of Nutrition
School of Public Health
Harvard University

OBJECTIVES

To serve as a brief review of important issues in the science of nutrition

To illustrate how knowledge about nutrition applies to solving certain
problems in contemporary medicine and health

To stimulate the reader's interest in learning more about nutrition

Baird A. Thomas

Editor Emeritus

Library of Congress Card Number 71:112745

Fourth Edition

The Upjohn Company, Kalamazoo, Michigan

MS 7630E

Contents

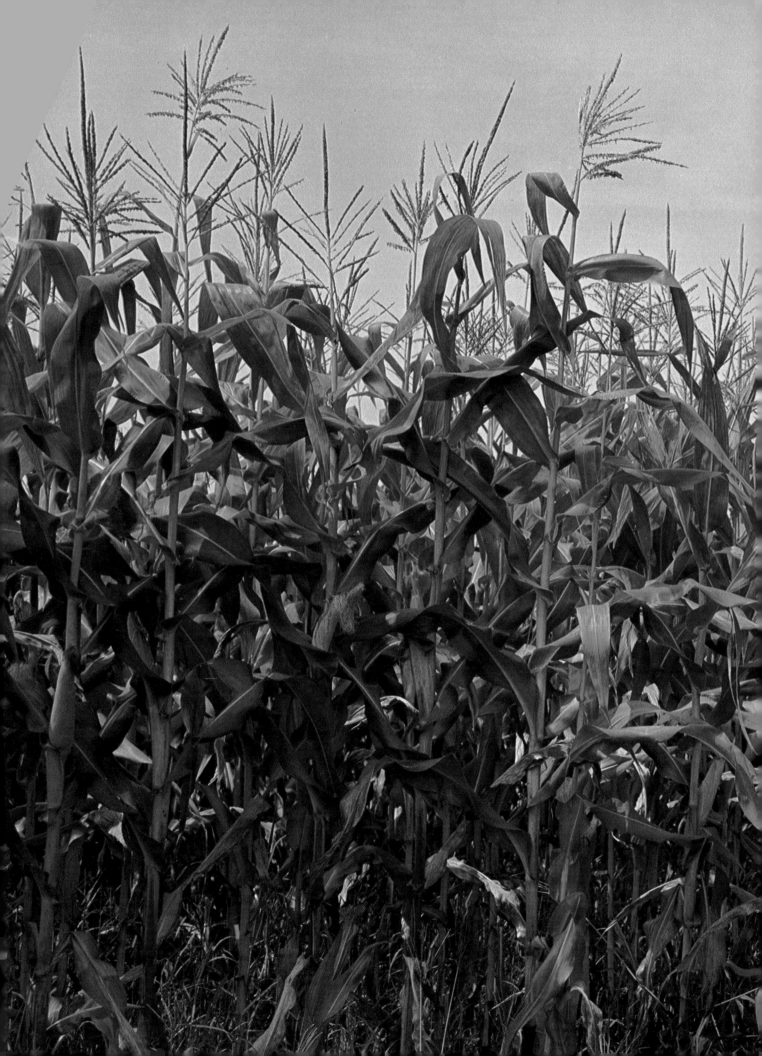

Preface

Fredrick J. Stare, MD
Professor of Nutrition
Founder and Former Chairman
Department of Nutrition
School of Public Health
Harvard University

Our primary job has been, and is, teaching, training, research-ing, and sending "our products" elsewhere to teach, train, research, and be of service in nutrition, which we consider an important and a largely neglected field of health and med-icine. When the idea, and then the first draft, of this Manual on Nutrition was born, my three original collaborators were all young physician-nutritionists, members of Harvard's Department of Nutrition. But before this Manual was com-pleted, two of my associates had left us. Dr. Michael Latham is now Professor of International Nutrition at Cornell Univer-sity in Ithaca, New York; and Dr. Mary B. McCann, having held a position of high responsibility in the United States Public Health Service ten-state nutrition surveys, became Professor of Nutrition, Department of Health Sciences, at Boston University. She is now a resident in psychiatry at Maine Medical Center in Portland. I am indebted to both of them for their help, particularly Dr. Latham who has always done more than his share.

Dr. Robert B. McGandy was an Associate Professor of Nutri-tion with us and played an important role in the preparation of the final draft for the first printing of this Manual. But he also has left our department and is now Professor of Nutrition and Clinical Professor of Pathology at Tufts University. Other members or former members of Harvard's Department of Nutrition – Drs. D. S. Bernstein, Phin Cohen, Robert P. Geyer, K. C. Hayes, D. M. Hegsted, George R. Kerr, Bernard Lown, Martha Singer, and Jelia Witschi have had a hand in either writing or reading various sections of this Manual.

In this fourth edition, which contains several new sections, Dr. Mohamed el Lozy, a relatively new member of the depart-ment, and Dr. M. Guillermo Herrera have played more-active roles and hence join us as co-authors.

We all hope this Manual, which is not a textbook, not a reference book, but a manual on nutrition primarily for med-ical, dental, and other health students, house officers, and practitioners of medicine and dentistry, will teach a little nutrition and stimulate considerable interest in learning more nutrition and its application to problems of contem-porary medicine and health.

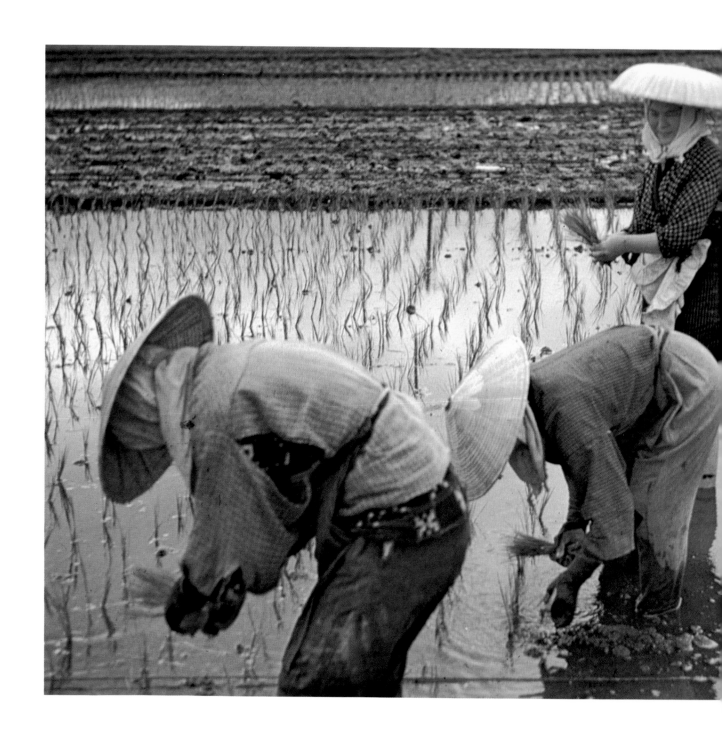

Introduction

Proper nutrition is an important factor in health, and malnutrition is an important factor in the etiology of several of the major causes of death and disability in our contemporary society. Atherosclerotic vascular disease, hypertension, obesity, tooth decay, osteoporosis, diabetes, and cancer are common diseases in which nutrition is closely involved.

In the developing areas of the world, some of the greatest health problems are directly related to inadequate nutrition. These include early childhood malnutrition due to calorie-protein deficiencies as well as iodine deficiency goiter, blindness due to lack of vitamin A, and a host of infectious diseases made worse by poor nutrition.

Iron-deficiency anemia and dental caries, widespread disorders related to malnutrition, have neither geographic nor socioeconomic boundaries. Even in highly developed societies there may be large segments of the population in which hunger and undernutrition impair physical and mental performance.

When the first edition of this Manual was published, instruction in the principles and practice of proper nutrition was almost nonexistent in most of our medical, dental, public health, and nursing schools. The biochemical and physiological basis of nutrition was frequently not a part of the preclinical sciences. Clinically, the major emphasis had been placed more on drugs and surgery than on the nutritional aspects of management, and almost no attention was paid to the role of nutrition in the prevention of illness and the improvement of health.

Fortunately, the situation has changed for the better. Nutrition is taught today in most of our professional schools. We like to think that this Manual has contributed to that change. More than 100,000 copies of the first three editions have been distributed to medical students not only in the United States but also throughout the world. We do know that many of our former students have played a prominent part in the awakening of interest in teaching nutrition.

Nutrition is the science of food, the materials or nutrients in food, what they do and how they interact – all in relation to health. Nutrition comes from food, good food that one enjoys (for eating has always been one of the pleasures of life), from food in variety so as to supply the more than 50 known nutrients that are necessary for proper nutrition, thereby providing the best of health that one's genetic or hereditary background permits. This manual includes four beautiful, colored pictures of farm scenes to emphasize that good nutrition comes from agriculture – that is, from foods provided by farmers.

Variety in foods consumed is the keystone to proper nutrition, because no single food provides all the known nutrients – not even mothers' milk. Consuming no more calories than required to reach and maintain a desirable body weight is also important. This depends in large part on one's physical activities, because muscular activities are the only way one has of using up calories beyond those needed for basal metabolism, doing a job well, and whatever one does with leisure or spare time. Maintenance of a desirable body weight also depends on attention to portion size, that is, how much one eats and drinks. A six-ounce steak provides twice the calories of a three-ounce steak, of course, and so do two glasses of beer as compared with one.

In the past decade or so, it has been found that the caloric balance, the type of fat in the diet, as well as the cholesterol content of the diet are important factors affecting the level of cholesterol in the blood. The latter is one of the factors (and a most important one) in affecting susceptibility to coronary heart disease and cerebral hemorrhage. The higher the level of cholesterol (and also other fats) in the blood, the greater the chances of developing these common causes of death, particularly when hypercholesterolemia occurs in association with other conditions such as elevated blood pressure, family history of cardiovascular-related premature death, cigarette smoking, diabetes mellitus, overweight, lethargy, or infrequent physical activity.

Nutrition as a science can be regarded as the study of six main categories of food components: protein, carbohydrate, fat, minerals, vitamins, and water. The first three categories – protein, carbohydrate, and fat – are the only ones that provide calories. Protein provides 4 Calories/gm, as does carbohydrate. Fat provides slightly more than twice as much – 9 Calories/gm.

Alcohol is not considered a foodstuff, but from time immemorial it has been consumed in various fermented and distilled beverages, and it does supply about 7 Calories/gm, so it must be considered in evaluating one's total caloric intake.

Although minerals and vitamins provide no calories, they function in the many metabolic processes whereby one obtains and utilizes energy from foods and builds and then maintains body tissues. Minerals also function as vital constituents of many body tissues. Iron is a necessary component of hemoglobin, myoglobin, and the cytochromes, and calcium and fluoride are required for sound teeth and bones.

Water, in addition to making up nearly 70% of the total body, is essential for the absorption of many nutrients, the elimination of body wastes via the urine and feces, and the maintenance of a normal body temperature by means of evaporation of water from the lungs and skin. Although water provides no calories or vitamins, "hard" water provides calcium and magnesium, and when fluoridated, either naturally or artificially, water is the only important source of the mineral nutrient fluoride. This mineral nutrient is not only the single most important factor in lessening tooth decay (by 60% to 70%) but also is important in lessening the incidence of osteoporosis in aging, and it may be important in lessening the incidence and severity of soft-tissue calcification as, for example, in hardening of the arteries.

Nutrition is important in modern health and medicine – in improving and maintaining good health and in improving poor health. It is hoped that this manual will stimulate students as well as practitioners of the health professions – medicine, dentistry, public health, and nursing – to learn more about nutrition and apply it for the benefit of mankind.

How prevalent is malnutrition in the United States?

This depends in part on what we mean by malnutrition. If we mean illness or poor health resulting in part from poor nutrition, it is widespread and occurs among all economic classes. For here we would include tooth decay due to inadequate intake of the mineral nutrient fluoride: tooth decay is almost universal. We would include osteoporosis contributed to by lack of fluoride, a condition that is radiologically demonstrable in 50% of adults over 60 years of age.

Related in part to malnutrition is atherosclerosis as manifested by coronary heart disease, cerebral, renal, and peripheral artery disease. Essential hypertension can be lessened by decreasing the intake of the mineral nutrient sodium, and may possibly be caused by too much sodium and aggravated by obesity. These cardiovascular diseases are responsible for well over half the deaths in this country. Iron-deficiency anemia is certainly prevalent in all societies. Certain types of cancer also appear to be associated with improper nutrition.

The acute and severe vitamin deficiencies as manifested by the classical nutritional diseases – scurvy, pellagra, beriberi, and xerophthalmia – are now uncommon in the United States, but they are prevalent in many other parts of the world. Vitamin deficiencies, however, are prevalent in a large number of alcoholics in our country.

We have few data to determine whether mild deficiencies of vitamins or other nutrients (particularly the trace minerals) are prevalent in the United States and particularly whether they are responsible for manifestations of ill health.

Extensive nutritional surveys to evaluate health in relation to nutrient intake have been completed in ten states.[1] It is important that techniques for such studies be improved. The studies should be extended to consider more nutrients and to provide factual data on the extent of malnutrition, not only among underprivileged people but also among privileged, and especially among young children. There should be continued monitoring of the nutritional status of representative groups of our people. Infant mortality rates in the United States are higher than in many other nations; we do not know the contribution of malnutrition to these deaths, but we do know that the death rates are higher among minority groups whose diets tend to be poor.

Clearly, there is something wrong with our food distribution system. In the same city it is quite common to find school meals provided in the affluent suburbs but not in the ghetto sections. Food stamps are sometimes available, but frequently the money to buy the stamps is not. Surplus food distribution has been designed much more to help the producer of surplus foods than the poverty-stricken consumer. Fortunately, the situation is improving.

We do not know how often an empty belly leads individual Americans into crime or what the contribution of anxiety is to violence and rioting among people having insufficient food. We do not yet know the role that malnutrition plays in mental and behavioral development of children.

We do know that all is not well nutritionally in this most affluent of nations. Improved nutrition allied with other measures of health and social justice can make America a better place for all her citizens. We can and must solve the problems of overnutrition – of too many calories, of too much cholesterol and saturated fat – in the affluent and of nutritional deficiencies and varying degrees of starvation in the poor, the alcoholics, the aged, the senile, and the dejected.

Interest in nutrition as an important environmental factor in the health of man is increasing rapidly. This stems from many directions, such as the realization that tooth decay, one of our most prevalent diseases, can be reduced by half or more by adjusting (usually upward) the content of the mineral nutrient fluoride in community waters, a process known as fluoridation; that lowering the cholesterol level of the blood lessens the chances of developing coronary heart disease or a stroke; that essential hypertension can frequently be treated simply by a modest loss of weight and a generous decrease in the intake of sodium; and that iron-deficiency anemia, prevalent in about one fourth of our total population, can usually be corrected simply by adding iron to the diet. It is a noted fact that obesity is widely prevalent in our country. Obesity by itself, when only moderate, may not be a health hazard, yet it seldom exists by itself and therefore is a real hazard to health. Finally, we know now that undernutrition as a partner of poverty is far more prevalent than had been expected.

But here too, progress has been made in recent years (and months), stemming largely from the White House Conference on Food and Nutrition. The conference, held in Washington, DC, in early December of 1969, was organized by Professor Jean Mayer, then of Harvard's Department of Nutrition, ably assisted by other members of this department. The Conference recommended a number of measures that have since been implemented, at least to some extent:

1 The Food-Stamp program has been made more widely available, allowing more food at reduced costs to the needy. Food stamps are provided without charge to those with no resources.

2 The Commodities program has been improved to provide for more-balanced diets by increasing the number of commodities given each month to the needy.

3 The Meals-on-Wheels and Community Meals for the Elderly programs have been expanded by federal assistance to state, local, and private projects that provide nutritional support for the aged and disabled.

4 The School Lunch Program has been expanded to provide lunches (and, in some cases, breakfasts) for millions of children who might otherwise have no food during the school day.

5 Pregnant and nursing women have been encouraged, educated, and helped to obtain more-nutritious foods.

6 The food-production industry and regulatory agencies have cooperated in a variety of measures to encourage proper nutrition. Expiration-dating of perishable foods, unit pricing, nutritional labeling, and continued research on the safety of food additives have permitted consumers a more active role in selecting nutritious and economical foods.

7 Various private and governmental programs have provided for increased nutritional education for both professional and lay people.

The Congress has recently stimulated considerable interest in nutrition, primarily through the establishment of the Senate Select Committee on Nutrition, which, since January of 1978, has been a part of the larger Committee on Agriculture. Although some of the Select Committee's reports have been quite controversial (particularly the so-called Dietary Goals), the Committee has nevertheless stirred up considerable interest in nutrition among the Congress, the public, and health-care professionals.

This manual is not a textbook of nutrition. It is intended simply to illustrate how nutrition relates to the health of mankind. For that reason, we have not discussed in any detail the many diseases in which dietary factors are particularly important. Excellent textbooks and other materials are available on nutritional management of the diabetic patient, for example, and the student should refer to them. But we hope he or she will do so with more intense interest and greater appreciation for having read this manual.

Recommended Dietary Allowances of Nutrients

This manual has been prepared primarily for use by medical students and physicians in the United States. Following is part of the introduction to the publication *Recommended Dietary Allowances*,[2] which is a report of the Food and Nutrition Board, National Academy of the Sciences-National Research Council of the United States (Table I). The publication provides the recommended daily dietary allowances of nutrients ("RDA") and gives an explanation of how these allowances are estimated.

"Since 1940, the Food and Nutrition Board has developed formulations of daily nutrient intakes which were judged to be adequate for the maintenance of good nutrition in the population of the United States. These formulations were designated 'Recommended Dietary Allowances' in order to indicate that they were value judgments based on the existing knowledge of nutritional science and subject to revision as new knowledge became available. The allowances are intended to serve as goals toward which to aim in planning food supplies and as guides for the interpretation of food consumption records of groups of people. Actual nutritional status of groups of people or individuals must be judged on the basis of physical, biochemical, and clinical observations combined with observations on food or nutrient intakes. If the recommended allowances are used as reference standards for interpreting records of food consumption, it should not be assumed that food practices are necessarily poor or that malnutrition exists because the recommendations are not completely met.

"The first edition of Recommended Dietary Allowances was published in 1943. The allowances recommended are those which, in the opinion of the Food and Nutrition Board, will maintain good nutrition in essentially *all* healthy persons in the United States under current conditions of living.

"The physiological and biochemical bases for the recommended allowances of each specific nutrient are described in the text. For proper understanding, application, and interpretation of the recommended allowances, it is necessary to appreciate how the allowances are related to estimates of average physiological requirements.

"The allowances are designed to afford a margin of sufficiency above average physiological requirements to cover variations among essentially all individuals in the general population. They provide a buffer against the increased needs during common stresses and permit full realization of growth and productive potential, but they are not to be considered adequate to meet additional requirements of persons depleted by disease or traumatic stresses. On the other hand, the allowances are generous with respect to temporary emergency feeding of large groups under conditions of limited food supply and physical disaster.

"The margin of sufficiency above normal physiological requirements is different for each nutrient because of differences in the body storage capacity, in the range of individual requirements, in the precision of assessing requirements, and in the possible hazard of excessive intake of certain nutrients. "Patterns of food consumption and food supplies in the United States permit ready adaptation to and compliance with the recommended allowances. The final objective of the recommended allowances is to permit and to encourage the development of food practices by the population of the United States that will allow for greatest dividends in health and in disease prevention."

The Recommended Dietary Allowances therefore provide guidelines for the evaluation and development of diets for people in the United States. One should clearly understand that the values presented are not requirements, since many individuals are known to consume smaller amounts than those listed and still enjoy good health. On the other hand, it is recognized that the actual requirement for any nutrient is not precisely known, and the estimates of requirements always demonstrate rather large differences in various experiments and among various persons. The cause of these variations is generally unknown. No doubt they are explained partially by technical differences or errors of measurement and partially by actual differences in individual requirements, which may be of genetic origin. When the true requirement is unknown, there is safety in recommending levels of nutrient intake above the estimated minimal need. The Recommended Dietary Allowances therefore must not be considered actual requirements but rather levels of intake that should be entirely adequate for essentially all members of the population. This kind of dietary guidance seems appropriate in an affluent country such as the United States. It may not be appropriate in many parts of the world where more-urgent problems exist and where food and money are more-limiting factors for many people.

The presentation of one figure as a recommended intake for a particular group (as in Table I) is likely to be somewhat misleading and is often misinterpreted. The publication from which it is taken[3] provides explanations and justifications for values presented. The text should be consulted by those who are using the Table.

It should be pointed out that the Recommended Dietary Allowances in the various editions are not and never have been the same as the old Minimum Daily Requirements set forth by the Food and Drug Administration. The latter were usual many years ago in an attempt to actually maintain minimum daily requirements. They are now completely out of date, and there is no evidence to justify their continued use.

Table I

**Food and Nutrition Board, National Academy of Sciences – National Research Council
Recommended Daily Dietary Allowances,[a] Revised 1980**
Designed for the maintenance of good nutrition of practically all healthy people in the U.S.A.

	Age (years)	Weight (kg)	Weight (lb)	Height (cm)	Height (in)	Protein (gm)	Fat-Soluble Vitamins		
							Vitamin A (μg RE)[b]	Vitamin D (μg)[c]	Vitamin E (mg α TE)[d]
Infants	0.0-0.5	6	13	60	24	kg × 2.2	420	10	3
	0.5-1.0	9	20	71	28	kg × 2.0	400	10	4
Children	1-3	13	29	90	35	23	400	10	5
	4-6	20	44	112	44	30	500	10	6
	7-10	28	62	132	52	34	700	10	7
Males	11-14	45	99	157	62	45	1,000	10	8
	15-18	66	145	176	69	56	1,000	10	10
	19-22	70	154	177	70	56	1,000	7.5	10
	23-50	70	154	178	70	56	1,000	5	10
	51+	70	154	178	70	56	1,000	5	10
Females	11-14	46	101	157	62	46	800	10	8
	15-18	55	120	163	64	46	800	10	8
	19-22	55	120	163	64	44	800	7.5	8
	23-50	55	120	163	64	44	800	5	8
	51+	55	120	163	64	44	800	5	8
Pregnant						+30	+200	+5	+2
Lactating						+20	+400	+5	+3

a The allowances are intended to provide for individual variations among most normal persons as they live in the United States under usual environmental stresses. Diets should be based on a variety of common foods in order to provide other nutrients for which human requirements have been less well defined.

b Retinol equivalents. 1 Retinol equivalent = 1 μg retinol or 6 μg carotene.

c As cholecalciferol. 10 μg cholecalciferol = 400 IU vitamin D.

d α tocopherol equivalents. 1 mg d-α-tocopherol = 1 αTE.

Water-Soluble Vitamins							Minerals					
Vitamin C (mg)	Thiamin (mg)	Riboflavin (mg)	Niacin (mg NE)[e]	Vitamin B_6 (mg)	Folacin[f] (μg)	Vitamin B_{12} (μg)	Calcium (mg)	Phosphorus (mg)	Magnesium (mg)	Iron (mg)	Zinc (mg)	Iodine (μg)
35	0.3	0.4	6	0.3	30	0.5[g]	360	240	50	10	3	40
35	0.5	0.6	8	0.6	45	1.5	540	360	70	15	5	50
45	0.7	0.8	9	0.9	100	2.0	800	800	150	15	10	70
45	0.9	1.0	11	1.3	200	2.5	800	800	200	10	10	90
45	1.2	1.4	16	1.6	300	3.0	800	800	250	10	10	120
50	1.4	1.6	18	1.8	400	3.0	1200	1200	350	18	15	150
60	1.4	1.7	18	2.0	400	3.0	1200	1200	400	18	15	150
60	1.5	1.7	19	2.2	400	3.0	800	800	350	10	15	150
60	1.4	1.6	18	2.2	400	3.0	800	800	350	10	15	150
60	1.2	1.4	16	2.2	400	3.0	800	800	350	10	15	150
50	1.1	1.3	15	1.8	400	3.0	1200	1200	300	18	15	150
60	1.1	1.3	14	2.0	400	3.0	1200	1200	300	18	15	150
60	1.1	1.3	14	2.0	400	3.0	800	800	300	18	15	150
60	1.0	1.2	13	2.0	400	3.0	800	800	300	18	15	150
60	1.0	1.2	13	2.0	400	3.0	800	800	300	10	15	150
+20	+0.4	+0.3	+2	+0.6	+400	+1.0	+400	+400	+150	h	+5	+25
+40	+0.5	+0.5	+5	+0.5	+100	+1.0	+400	+400	+150	h	+10	+50

e 1 NE (niacin equivalent) is equal to 1 mg of niacin or 60 mg of dietary tryptophan.

f The folacin allowances refer to dietary sources as determined by *Lactobacillus casei* assay after treatment with enzymes ("conjugases") to make polyglutamyl forms of the vitamin available to the test organism.

g The RDA for vitamin B_{12} in infants is based on average concentration of the vitamin in human milk. The allowances after weaning are based on energy intake (as recommended by the American Academy of Pediatrics) and consideration of other factors such as intestinal absorption.

h The increased requirement during pregnancy cannot be met by the iron content of habitual American diets nor by the existing iron stores of many women; therefore the use of 30-60 mg of supplemental iron is recommended. Iron needs during lactation are not substantially different from those of nonpregnant women, but continued supplementation of the mother for 2-3 months after parturition is advisable in order to replenish stores depleted by pregnancy.

Nutritional Aspects of
Selected Medical Problems

NUTRITIONAL CONCEPTS IN HEART DISEASE
The Use of Nutrition in the Prevention
of Atherosclerotic Cardiovascular Disease

Atherosclerotic vascular disease involving the coronary and cerebral circulation is the leading cause of death in the United States today. The disabilities among survivors of myocardial and cerebral infarction comprise problems of enormous magnitude concerning the socioeconomic and medical aspects of individual care. Coronary heart disease is more frequent among men in the fourth and fifth decades of life. The magnitude of the problem of atherosclerosis (which begins in the second decade of life in overnourished societies) and the premature mortality associated with coronary heart disease demand large-scale preventive measures to reduce overall incidence and death rates.[4] Current medical practice cannot significantly mitigate morbidity and mortality from these causes.

Present concepts of atherosclerotic vascular disease suggest that a number of environmental influences interact with host factors in progression of the disease and its ultimate clinical manifestations. It is quite apparent that this disease is not the inevitable consequence of either age or hereditary tendencies per se. Comprehensive evaluation of the evidence from clinical, pathological, epidemiological, and experimental animal studies suggests multifactorial causation. Diet, through its influence on lipid metabolism and circulating lipids, is an important environmental element. Other factors associated with coronary heart disease are hypertension, cigarette smoking, adiposity, and physical inactivity. The latter two are clearly interrelated. Resolution and understanding of the contributions and interactions of these factors as related to accelerated, premature clinical manifestations of atherosclerotic vascular disease have proved unhappily difficult. Even the extensive descriptive population studies cannot provide all the answers. Ultimate cellular and biochemical mechanisms are obscure. An adequate experimental animal model for the investigation of atherosclerosis and its clinical sequelae in man is not available.

Of all the basic regulating factors known to be associated with the disease and that can be realistically manipulated to prevent or at least retard the atherosclerotic process, nutrition stands out. Elevation of the blood-lipid concentration, particularly the induction of hyperbetalipoproteinemia, is mandatory for the experimental induction of atherosclerosis in animals. Dietary manipulation is the easiest way to achieve

experimental atherogenesis. The extraordinary differences in blood lipids among peoples of various areas of the world are correlated with cardiovascular disease mortality. Differences in lipid distributions are related to dietary practices. The association of accelerated development of atherosclerosis and coronary heart disease with metabolic disorders in which circulating lipid concentrations are elevated has long been recognized. A major contribution of the large, descriptive, epidemiologic study has been the demonstration of a quantitative association between lipids and the subsequent incidence of coronary and thrombotic cerebrovascular disease. The relationship shown in Figure 1 is typical of the association found in population studies.

To demonstrate relationships between factors and specific disease does not prove unique causality. The only proper way to identify causality in man is to carry out a controlled clinical trial designed to assess risk of disease in an appropriately sampled group in whom a factor associated with risk has been manipulated. A suitable study design, properly controlled, is mandatory.

Of all the factors related to atherosclerotic vascular diseases aside from controlling hypertension (even mild hypertension), dietary changes to reduce blood lipids are more practical and effective than is intervention in other risk factors, considering the lamentable status of our ability to motivate people to alter their life-style. Persistent weight reduction, alteration of smoking habits, and changing patterns of physical activity are very difficult to achieve in most persons. Today there is increasingly secure evidence from clinical trials that dietary changes aimed at reducing the levels of serum lipids, especially cholesterol, can significantly reduce the incidence of coronary heart disease in man. One of the early controlled trials,[5] in a study of men who had survived a myocardial infarction, showed that the group treated with a lipid-controlled diet had a significantly reduced incidence of myocardial reinfarction and angina pectoris over a five-year follow-up period as compared to the counterpart control group. The average reduction in serum cholesterol in the diet-controlled groups was 17%.

That study and many more-recent studies demonstrate that diet is an important regulator of the plasma proteins, which, in human beings, are closely associated with atherosclerosis and with the variety of clinical manifestations of the process – coronary heart disease, thrombotic cerebrovascular disease, occlusive peripheral vascular disease, and aortic aneurysm. Thus, it seems reasonable to assume that dietary modifications leading to more-favorable concentrations of plasma lipoproteins would lead to less atherosclerosis.

We do know that over the past few years there has been a significant decrease in death rates from atherosclerotic diseases in the American population. We do not know how much of that decrease can be ascribed to changes in the diet, to changes in other "life-style" factors (exercise, weight control, smoking habits), to effective pharmacologic management of hypertension, or to improved treatment of acute disease in coronary care units.

Nevertheless, persuasive arguments for a preventive approach to atherosclerotic vascular disease, ideally beginning in childhood and adolescence, are based upon the following facts:

1 Atherosclerosis is an essentially universal disease among Americans from the second decade of life. The differences among us are in the extent, severity, and locations of the process. The underlying disease thus precedes clinical manifestations by 20 to 50 years.

2 Therapeutic measures aimed at ameliorating the atherosclerotic process are clearly less reliable in advanced lesions that are complicated by fibrosis and calcification. The best direct evidence for the reversibility of atherosclerosis comes from several studies with primates. Concentrations of low-density plasma lipoproteins were elevated by feeding the animals a "typical American" diet high in saturated fats and cholesterol. The result was atherosclerosis characterized by fatty streaks and fibromuscular plaques identical to that seen in young adult humans. When the monkeys were returned to their normal diet, the lesions regressed.

Epidemiologic studies, whether carried out in the United States (the well-known Framingham Study, for example) or in any other of the many industrialized countries, have consistently demonstrated an association between the plasma concentrations of low-density lipoproteins (most easily assessed by measuring total cholesterol) and vascular diseases. The plasma cholesterol concentration of the average middle-aged American male is 240 mg/dl. Men of the same age who have plasma cholesterol values of 200 mg/dl are only half as likely to have coronary heart disease, and those whose values are 270 mg/dl or greater have more than twice the "average" risk. As previously stated, other risk factors have also been identified: elevated blood pressure, cigarette smoking, diabetes, obesity, and perhaps others. More recently it has been

Figure 1A. Relative risks of developing coronary heart disease, according to initial serum cholesterol levels. Men initially aged 30-59 years and followed up for ten years.

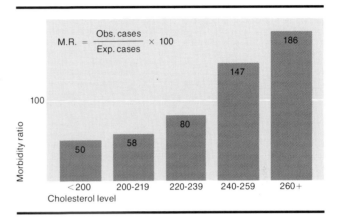

Figure 1B. Prevalence and mortality of cerebrovascular disease (CVD).

Prevalence[*]
26,634,000 Americans have some form of heart and blood vessel disease (excluding varicose veins, hemorrhoids, and phlebitis):

hypertension	23,171,000
coronary heart disease	3,307,000
disorders of heart rhythm	2,442,000
cerebrovascular disease	1,534,000

Mortality[**]
CVD mortality – 974,429 (51% of all deaths)
21.8% of all persons killed by CVD are under age 65.

acute myocardial infarction	319,477
chronic ischemic heart disease	322,382
cerebrovascular disease	188,623
hypertension and related	25,910
arteriosclerosis	29,366
other CVD	88,671

Comparative Mortality Data[**]
Cancer   377,317 (20% of all deaths)
Accidents 100,761
All other   456,938

[*]Prevalence data from NCHS, Vital and Health Statistics, series 10, number 94 – Prevalence of chronic circulatory conditions, United States, 1972, except for hypertension from Advance Data from Vital and Health Statistics, number 7, October 18, 1976.
[**]Mortality data from Monthly Vital Statistics Report, Advance Report. Final Mortality Statistics for 1976.

learned that another class of lipoproteins (the high-density class) is relatively protective against atherosclerosis. How this category is influenced by diet, exercise, and diabetes remains to be learned.

Although there is much that we still do not know about atherosclerosis, and in particular about how diet and lipids are ultimately related to the disease process, that should not obscure what we do know. Atherosclerosis is not inevitably present among human populations, it is not an inevitable concomitant of aging, and it cannot be accounted for on the basis of genetic factors alone. Environmental influences are of the greatest importance.

The aims of dietary management to reduce serum cholesterol concentrations are to:

a Adjust the caloric balance to ensure a desirable body weight, generally by moderately restricting caloric intake and increasing physical activity.

b Decrease the intake of saturated fat, which, in the usual diet, is from meats and dairy products. The patient should be encouraged to trim fat from carefully selected meat and to consume smaller portions. Fish and poultry contain lesser quantities of total and saturated fats than do other meats and should therefore be emphasized in the diet. Low-fat dairy products can be substituted for their high-fat counterparts, and high-fat baked products should be avoided unless the fat is polyunsaturated.

c Reduce the intake of dietary cholesterol. The usual daily consumption of 600 to 800 mg of cholesterol can be reduced to half by limiting the use of egg yolks to two or three a week. The consumption of lean meats and low-fat dairy products in preference to organ meats (such as liver), fatty meats (such as pork), and high-fat dairy products (such as butter and cream) will also help to limit the intake of cholesterol.

d Increase the intake of polyunsaturated fats, which are abundant in corn, soya, safflower, sunflower, and cottonseed oils. Used as cooking and salad oils and as margarine and shortening (with a minimum of hydrogenation), they can substitute for animal fat, thereby reducing the serum cholesterol concentration while permitting a palatable diet.

Persons who follow those dietary guidelines can expect to reduce the proportion of fats in the caloric balance from the usual 40% to 45% to about 35% to 40%. The ratio of polyunsaturated fat to saturated fat will then be about 1:1 or greater.

Note on circulating lipids: The plasma lipoproteins (complexes of triglyceride, cholesterol, phospholipid, and protein) are the agents most closely associated with atherosclerosis. The concentrations of circulating lipoproteins can be estimated by measuring the total plasma cholesterol and the fasting triglyceride concentrations. Knowledge of the patient's plasma cholesterol value alone is sufficient for screening and assessing management in most of the population, but about 5% of middle-aged persons have either plasma cholesterol values of at least 300 mg/dl or a lactescent fasting serum, or both. In treating or evaluating such a patient, determination of lipoprotein electrophoretic or physicochemical properties is important.[6]

The lipoproteins are classified as Very Low Density (VLDL, or pre β), Low Density (LDL, or β), and High Density (HDL, or α). The development of atherosclerosis is associated more closely with LDL than with HDL, which in fact may have a protective effect.[7] Thus, there may be "good cholesterol" (HDL) and "bad cholesterol" (LDL); many investigators are therefore attempting to determine the factors that influence the relative concentrations of the lipoproteins.

Hypertension and Congestive Heart Failure

Reduction of body sodium by dietary restriction and pharmacologic intervention are the aims of current nutritional therapy for heart failure and hypertension. Net body loss of sodium in the person with a failing heart reduces extracellular fluid volume, thereby correcting edema and its complications and reducing circulating fluid volume, all of which lessens the work of the heart. The resulting improvement of organ perfusion, especially of the kidneys, results in the ability of intrinsic homeostatic mechanisms to regain control of sodium balance and improves exercise tolerance.

Today's physician is becoming increasingly aware that the natriuretic drugs, the diuretics and cardiac glycosides, are not without hazard, and, lamentably, not infrequently have had fatal consequences. Effective diuretics are associated with the loss of potassium as well as sodium. Potassium depletion secondary to diuretic therapy increases myocardial irritability and predisposes the patient to threatening arrhythmias. This compromise is potentiated by the cardiac glycosides, drugs used frequently in combination with the potassium-depleting diuretics. Too frequently, drugs are employed in the treatment of patients who would respond to dietary sodium restriction alone if it were prescribed with the same conviction.

The aim of nutritional therapy is to induce negative sodium balance in the body. The physician prescribes a diet that is adequate nutritionally but restricted in its sodium content. In the United States, the usual daily intake of sodium ion is about 3 to 7 gm, or 150 to 300 mEq. The sodium content of therapeutic regimens ranges from 2.3 gm (100 mEq) per day in the "no-added-salt" diet to as low as 230 mg (10 mEq).

Patients frequently misunderstand the sources of salt or sodium in the diet. It is the responsibility of the physician and the dietitian to ensure that the patient understands that some foods *naturally* contain sodium. The most understandable explanation is that just as we retain sodium in our bodies, so does the animal; foods of animal origin – meat, milk, cheese, and butter – are therefore major sources of dietary sodium. The processes of food preservation often necessitate the addition of salt, and thus many smoked, cured, and canned foods contain high concentrations of sodium. Many food condiments and flavor enhancers contain sodium in the form of monosodium glutamate (MSG). Food charts are available that provide information on the amount of sodium contained in common foods, expressed usually in milligrams (with 1 mEq equal to 23 mg of sodium ion [Appendix A]). (The American Heart Association can provide the physician with excellent materials for patient education.)

It is true that diuretics and cardiac glycosides are among our most potent therapeutic tools in dealing with a patient with heart failure, and they are definitely indicated in addition to dietary sodium restriction in the severely compromised patient. If there exists a clinical necessity for the use of these drugs together, or of the diuretics alone, potassium supplementation must be instituted. Potassium salts are gastric irritants and are unpalatable, causing nausea, vomiting, and rejection by the patient. This is why potassium salts have been given as enteric coated tablets. Enteric coated preparations, however, may cause ulceration of the small intestine, with unhappy consequences. If potassium supplementation is necessary, potassium-rich foods are an economical, palatable, and a simple approach contrasted with potassium elixirs. Especially with these preparations the possibility of overdosage must be considered, another probable fatal result of the failure to recognize the safer nutritional approach.

Diuretic-treated patients may need potassium ion intakes as high as 5 gm (130 mEq) per day. A list of foods that are good sources of potassium is found in Appendix A. The nutritional approach to sodium restriction and potassium supplementation cannot be understated as an important adjunct for the patient requiring manipulation of electrolyte balance.

In summarizing the role of dietary sodium in regulating blood pressure, one can state that 2.0 to 2.5 gm per day of sodium, an essential mineral nutrient, will adequately cover requirements among adults performing ordinary activities in temperate climates. Yet dietary surveys have shown that habitual intakes of sodium average two to five times that amount. Such excessive loads have been linked with hypertension in experimental animal studies and may be associated with hypertension in some human beings. Briefly, the evidence is as follows:

1 Sodium-restricted diets (0.1 to 0.5 gm per day) are usually effective in lowering essential hypertension in humans.

2 Populations that routinely consume very low levels of sodium show little or no increases in blood pressure throughout adult life (in contrast to the age-related increase in blood pressure seen in industrialized societies) and no "hypertension" by our criteria.

3 Dietary sodium is a regulator of blood pressure in certain strains of experimental animals.

What is not known is whether *moderate* restrictions of dietary sodium (to the 2 to 5 gm per day recommended in the US Dietary Goals) would in time lead to lower blood pressures and thus aid in the primary prevention of hypertension.

OBESITY

Forty-five percent of the adult American population are at least 20% above Desirable Weight and thus, by definition, obese. Obesity carries with it a substantial incremental risk of diabetes, coronary artery disease, hypertension, orthopedic problems, blood-lipid disorders, and eclampsia. It constitutes, therefore, one of the major health problems of industrialized countries. Figure 2 shows the excessive mortality attributable to obesity among young and middle-aged American adults. In only a fraction of a percent of cases can obesity be attributed to known metabolic disorders such as hypothyroidism.

Most human obesity remains a symptom of a homeostatic disorder of unknown nature. The obese are characterized by reduced physical activity and relentless weight gain through a combination of inappropriate intake of calories in relation to needs. A disorder of food-intake regulation is strongly suggested by the usual refractoriness to treatment (by most means so far tested) and by a very high recurrence rate among those who have successfully dieted. Thus, prevention of excessive weight gain is the best available approach to the problem.

20

Figure 2. Relation of body weight to mortality.

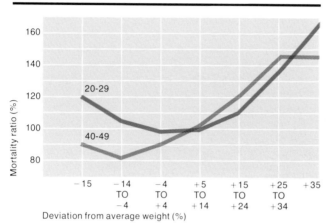

The death rate for deviations from the mean body weight has been plotted for persons aged 20 to 29 and 40 to 49. The 100 percent figure on the ordinate represents the number of deaths per 100,000 insured people of all weights in each age group. The deviations from this 100 percent figure represent greater or lesser numbers of deaths in the subgroups of the population whose deviations in body weight are plotted on the abscissa.

Adapted with permission from: Bray GA, Davidson MB, Drenick EJ: Obesity: A serious symptom. *Ann Intern Med* 77:779, 1972.

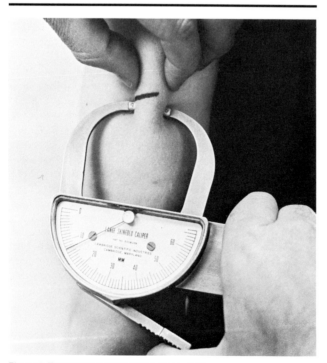

Figure 3. Triceps skinfold thickness measured by a skinfold caliper. Duplicate measurements should be obtained for an average measurement of adipose tissue.

Assessing Obesity

Obesity is defined as the excessive accumulation of adipose tissue fat as a result of caloric intake in excess of requirements for basal metabolism and physical activity. The terms "obesity" and "overweight" are not synonymous; the former denotes excessive adipose tissue, whereas the latter does not distinguish between body components – muscle, bone, and fat. A person may be overweight and yet not be obese – for example, a very muscular football player. Such cases among the general public are uncommon, however, and gross overweight usually implies gross obesity. Another factor that must be considered is fluid accumulation secondary to cardiovascular, renal, or hepatic disease or to less-well-understood causes such as occurs in cyclical edema. When retention of extracellular fluid exceeds 2 to 3 kg, it is usually detectable as edema or ascites.

Although total adipose tissue cannot be measured directly, the determination of skinfold thickness at standard sites does offer a simple method for quantitating adiposity. Such measurements are highly correlated with total body fat. Constant-pressure skinfold calipers make these measurements reliable. The triceps and subcapsular skinfolds are the sites generally used. The former is more accessible and gives reproducible results. With the patient's right arm flexed at 90°, a tape measure is used to accurately locate, on the back of the triceps, the midpoint between the tip of the acromion and the olecranon. A fold of skin pulled away at that site is then measured with the calipers (Figure 3). The upper limits of normal values for a healthy Caucasian American population are shown in Appendix F.

The use of height-weight tables remains the most practical method for quantitating overnutrition; their limitations have already been mentioned. The Tables of Desirable Weight (according to skeletal frame, size, and height) represent the weights of insurees with optimal life expectancy in a study done by the Society of Actuaries in 1959 (see Appendix D).

Excessive weight gain may occur at any stage of the life-span, but it tends to coincide with periods in which fat is normally accumulated at a faster pace: in infancy (if the child is overfed, particularly concentrated foods), during adolescence, and in pregnancy. Prevention should therefore receive priority at these times. It has been proposed but not proved that overfeeding during infancy may increase the total number of fat cells in the body. There is no doubt, however, that obesity that begins during childhood or adolescence is more difficult to control in later years. The steady increase in weight commonly noted after the third decade may be accounted for by a progressive decrease in physical activity and continued enjoyment of food.

Treatment and Prevention

Treatment of obesity has been generally unsuccessful. Dieting rarely achieves success, and, when it does, it is almost never long lasting. Anorectic drugs, notably amphetamines, may be effective appetite suppressors temporarily, but toxicity and the development of tolerance and dependency render them unsuitable for any role in the clinical management of obesity. Similarly ineffective has been the use of chorionic gonadotropin, growth hormone, and thyroid hormone. Psychotherapeutic methods have met with limited success, but newer approaches using behavior modification may be more successful. Intestinal bypass surgery is characterized by unpredictable results and serious complications. Obviously, much remains to be done in establishing the pathophysiology of obesity in order to develop effective treatment.

A competent medical evaluation; measurement of height, weight, and skinfold thickness; and an assessment of the patient's goals and motivation are needed to attempt treatment, and, more important, to plan preventive measures.

A proper therapeutic diet for obesity should provide all necessary nutrients in sufficient amounts and should be restricted in caloric content. It should be palatable, easily available, economical, and convenient. The patient should be educated so that once desired weight has been achieved, minor changes (such as increasing portion sizes) will provide a proper maintenance diet. The desired caloric deficit can be estimated, since a pound of body fat represents the equivalent of about 3500 Calories. Thus, a daily deficit of 500 Calories will result in an average weekly loss of one pound. In relatively active patients, a daily intake of less than 1500 Calories for men and 1000 for women is poorly tolerated. Increased physical activity can help increase the caloric deficit by 500 Calories per day without cutting food intake to this extent. Thus, a daily decrease of 300 Calories from food and drink and an increase in caloric expenditure of 200 Calories through exercise will be more acceptable to most people than would a total food caloric deficit of 500 Calories, yet will accomplish the same result.

Experience suggests that a balanced diet with 12% to 14% of calories as protein, 35% or less as fat (with a reduction in saturated fats) and the remaining calories supplied by carbohydrate is the best diet over a long period of time. There is no evidence that extreme "fad" diets have any advantage over a calorically restricted, balanced diet. Moreover, fad diets do not provide realistic behavior patterns that can be adopted for a lifetime. Some fad diets are actually dangerous to health as, for example, the "Zen Macrobiotic Diet" or the liquid hydrolized protein diets.

The chief advantage of "formula diets," which were popular a decade or more ago, is the provision of a simple, rigid regimen that does not need to be based on knowledge of food values. They may be useful at the beginning of a weight-control program or for a one-meal-a-day replacement in certain instances, but their use does not teach the patient good, long-term habits.

Bulk-producing agents such as methylcellulose have not been shown to have any merit. Salads, fruits, and vegetables are superior bulk-producing agents and are more palatable and more likely to become part of a lifelong dietary pattern.

Salt restriction is useful in those obese persons who have a tendency to retain fluid. Diuretics should be reserved for the treatment of edema.

Dessicated thyroid has been used as an adjunct to weight reduction on the grounds that obese patients are hypometabolic. Most obese patients, however, are euthyroid. Thyroid hormones in small doses suppress endogenous hormone production and therefore have no net effect. Larger doses produce hyperthyroidism with serious side effects. Thyroid tablets are therefore not recommended for use in weight-reduction programs.

Exercise is most important in a realistic reducing program. In most persons, reduction or elimination of exercise is not followed by a reduction in food intake. Conversely, exercise does not precipitate increased food intake in previously inactive persons until the physical activity reaches a certain critical duration and intensity. Behavior modification programs using group therapy have achieved better results than has one-to-one counseling by physicians or dietitians. Group members keep careful records of how much, where, and how food is consumed. The stimuli and cues associated with eating are identified, and techniques are developed to control excessive eating. Participants learn to reinforce the behaviors that result in reduced food intake. Continued interest and periodic supervision by the physician, dietitian, or group leader are essential for long-lasting control and prevention.

Obesity and Adult-Onset Diabetes Mellitus

Nutrition and diet play a significant role in the prevention and management of diabetes mellitus, which affects 5% of the U.S. population.

The relationship of obesity to the development of adult-onset diabetes deserves special emphasis.[8] Adult-onset diabetes is characterized by a relative lack of circulating insulin, accelerated atherosclerosis, and pathological changes in the blood vessels of the retina, kidney, and peripheral nerves. Heredity plays a role in the causation of the disease, but environmental factors determine its expression. Rates increase sharply with age and with the degree of obesity.

The incidence of diabetes has increased markedly in Africa, Israel, and Japan as those countries have adopted dietary patterns more consistent with those of the United States and as obesity has become more prevalent. Among some new-world populations, differences in the rates of diabetes as great as tenfold have been documented. The most important factors associated with the increased prevalence of diabetes are the degree and duration of obesity. Obesity has been shown to produce resistance to both exogenous and endogenous insulin. Refined sugars and fats have not been proved to be diabetogenic. Although a positive association has been found between consumption of sugar and fat and the prevalence of diabetes, the data suggest that they are not important risk factors apart from their possible effects on obesity. Weight reduction and exercise improve carbohydrate tolerance in nondiabetic and diabetic subjects. Dr. K. M. West[9] concludes: "A review of all available laboratory and epidemiological evidence suggests that the most important dietary factor in increasing the risk of diabetes is total calorie intake irrespective of source. This still leaves open the question regarding the importance of fat and sugar in inducing excessive caloric consumption."

The atherosclerotic complications of diabetes occur less frequently among populations that consume diets relatively low in cholesterol and saturated fats. Total caloric intake also plays an important role. It follows, therefore, that the single most important goal in the prevention and management of diabetes is control of total caloric intake to attain Desirable Weight. There is no need to restrict carbohydrates in the diets of most diabetic patients except to reduce the intake of refined and simple sugars (also honey), which include, mainly, sucrose and fructose. Reduction in cholesterol and restricted fat intake is also desirable. Here again, as in the management and prevention of obesity in the nondiabetic person, motivation and education of the patient and the community remain the major challenge for physicians, dietitians, nurses, and health educators.[10]

DENTAL CARIES

Dental caries is the most widespread disease in the United States. In some parts of the country, as many as 98% of the population surveyed have serious dental problems requiring either tooth extractions or restorations. A complete loss of teeth early in adolescence is occasionally seen and by middle age is fairly common. Edentulous persons often have difficulty in consuming certain foods and this sometimes makes it difficult for them to get a balanced diet. The dental profession does not have the trained manpower to provide adequate dental care for everyone. If poverty and lack of knowledge were not important factors in limiting the numbers seeking dental treatment, dentists would be overwhelmed and quite unable to cope with the dental pathology that would be presented to them. The prevention of dental caries by whatever means possible is therefore of great importance in public health.

Modern western diets and eating habits have clearly had an effect on the prevalence of dental caries, as is evident by surveys that demonstrate a much higher number of decayed, missing, and filled teeth among Americans as compared with groups of persons of the same age in many developing countries. Sticky adherent carbohydrate foods with a low rate of clearance from the oral cavity – particularly those foods eaten between meals – are almost certainly an important factor in this respect.[11]

Many nutrients are necessary for the development of the teeth and their surrounding structures. Vitamin A is important for normal bone growth. Inadequate growth patterns that result in orthodontic problems can result from vitamin A deficiency. The effects of a deficiency of vitamin C on the soft supporting tissues of the teeth are described on page 80. It should be noted that these gum lesions do not occur in edentulous persons. Protein is also essential for the normal development of the teeth and supporting tissues.

Vitamin D, calcium, and phosphorus, which are important in bone development, are also essential to the development of teeth. There is some controversy as to whether vitamin D supplementation helps to reduce caries susceptibility. The general balance of evidence suggests that where inadequate quantities of vitamin D are obtained either from the diet or

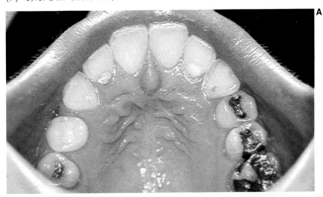

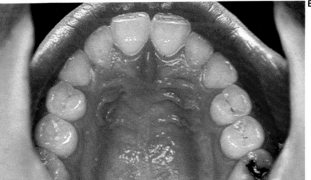

from exposure of the body to sunlight, vitamin D taken orally
will help to reduce the caries rate.

However, fluoride is the single most important mineral
nutrient in relation to dental caries (Figure 4). In the 1930s it
was observed that persons who had access to drinking water
that contained 1 to 2 parts per million (ppm) of fluoride had
considerably less tooth decay than did those whose water
supply had much lower amounts of fluoride. It was subsequently found that in areas where the water had very little
fluoride, it was possible to reduce the incidence of dental
caries by 60% to 70% by adjusting the fluoride level of the
water to about 1 ppm. In 1945, the first experimental study of
fluoride prophylaxis against dental caries was begun. Fluoride was added to the water in three communities – Newburgh,
New York; Brantford, Ontario; and Grand Rapids, Michigan.
Three neighboring cities with little or no fluoride in water
supplies were chosen as control communities. After ten years,
the rate of dental caries among children who had been consuming fluoridated water from an early age was 60% to 70%
lower than that of children in the control communities (Figures 5 and 6). Trials in other cities and in several countries
have shown similar results (Figures 7 and 8). The chemical
mechanism of fluoride's effect is now known, and today at
least 10,000 American communities of more than 120 million
people have fluoridated water.

There is no doubt that the fluoridation of water supplies
is a public health measure of very great importance. It is the
responsibility of every physician, dentist, and health worker
to urge and support fluoridation of the water supply where
needed. Generally, the opponents of fluoridation comprise
three categories: health faddists, those who for quasi-religious
reasons are opposed to any type of medication, and those
who equate fluoridation with an interference in their individual rights. Fluoridation has been found to be absolutely
safe at one part per million (ppm) for people of all ages and
in every state of health.[12,13] Fluoridation is not a form of medication, only an adjustment of the level of a nutrient, fluoride,
just as is the fortification of bread with vitamins. Fluoridation
is no more an infringement of freedom of individual rights
than is the chlorination of water or the regulation of the
speed limit.

There are substitutes for fluoridation, such as pills, drops,
and fluoridated toothpaste, but none combine the efficiency,
practicality, effectiveness, and economy of fluoridation for
the general public. The addition of fluoride to pediatric vita-

min preparations is very useful because fluoride has its maximum effectiveness when received early in life. Especially
when the infant is breast-fed, fluoride-vitamin supplements
are desirable, even where the water supply is fluoridated,
because fluoride does not readily cross the mammary gland
in adequate amounts.

For children fortunate to have been born and brought up in
communities where the water is fluoridated, the cost of "back-
log" dental care has been reduced by 60% and that of maintenance care by about 50%. With the constantly increasing costs
of health care, this is a most important economic factor.

Recent studies have shown that the fluoridation of drinking water in elementary and secondary schools to a level of
4.5 ppm will result in a reduction of caries by about 40%.
This higher level is required because children have access to
the water only during school hours and because they are five
to six years of age when they first begin to drink the fluoridated water.[14]

Figure 5. Reduction in decayed, missing, and filled permanent teeth (6- and 7-year-olds, 7 years after fluoridation).

City	PPM	% Reduction
Grand Rapids Michigan	1	61
Newburgh New York	1.1	69
Brantford Ontario, Canada	1	65

Dental examinations on 6- and 7-year-old children, seven years after the institution of fluoridation, have revealed a reduction of 61%, 69% and 65% in decayed, missing or filled teeth in Grand Rapids, Michigan; Newburgh, New York; and Brantford, Ontario, Canada, respectively.

Figure 6. Decayed, missing, and filled teeth* per child. Ten years after fluoridation.

*Permanent teeth

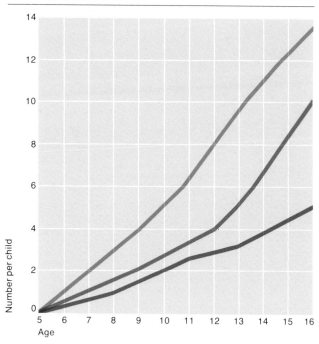

Grand Rapids, Michigan 1944 before fluoridation
Grand Rapids, Michigan 1954 10 years after fluoridation (1 ppm)
Aurora, Illinois 1945 naturally fluoridated water (1.2 ppm)

The rate of permanent-tooth caries in children who consumed fluoridated water since the time of birth was 60% to 70% less than that seen in children who did not receive fluoride.

Figure 7. Decayed, missing, and filled teeth of children 6-10 years old in fluoridated and non-fluoridated cities.

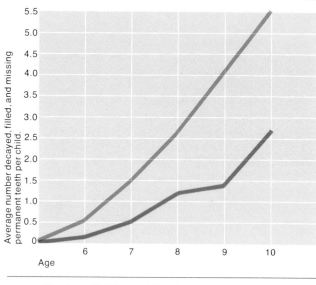

Kingston, N.Y., 0.0 ppm of fluoride
Newburgh, N.Y., 1.0-1.2 ppm of fluoride

Results from fluoridation in children 6-10 years old in Kingston, N.Y. (no fluoride) and Newburgh, N.Y. (1.0-1.2 ppm of fluoride).

Figure 8. Incidence of decayed and filled deciduous teeth (three years after first dental examination). Patient age approximately 7.

	Number of patients	% of children with all good teeth	Mean no. of new, decayed, and filled teeth
Infant Group (Fluoride-vitamin from birth)	108	60.2	0.98
Water Group (Fluoride in water from birth)	41	43.9	1.59
Baseline Group (Fluoride-vitamin since age 4)	277	30.3	2.14
Control Group (No fluoride)	212	24.5	2.92

Infants started on fluoride from birth compared to a control group showed more than twice as many children with all good teeth at age seven. These same groups showed approximately one filled tooth in the fluoride group for every three in the child who had no fluoride.

There is a statistical difference (P < .01) between the "control" and "infant" group and between the "infant" and "baseline" group (P + < .01) with the "infant" group having a statistically higher percentage of children with all good teeth.

P = probability.

Figure 9. Interaction of fluoride with the hydroxy-apatite mineral lattice of the teeth.

$$3 \cdot Ca_3P_2O_8 \cdot Ca\,(OH)_2 \quad \text{Hydroxyapatite}$$
$$+2F^- \qquad \text{(caries-susceptible)}$$
$$\downarrow$$
$$3\,Ca_3P_2O_8 \cdot Ca\,(F)_2 \quad \text{Fluorapatite}$$
$$+2\,OH^- \qquad \text{(promotes caries-resistance)}$$

OSTEOPOROSIS

Osteoporosis is a chronic disease of aging. It is extremely prevalent in the United States and is becoming ever more significant as the population tends to live longer.

The disease is characterized by excessive demineralization of bone, which is often responsible for considerable pain. Pain is common in the back and may radiate around the trunk and extend into the legs. The patient is sometimes incapacitated because the pain is aggravated by movement and by jarring the spine in walking. A frequent complication in the elderly is the fracturing of bones. This may be the collapse of one or more vertebrae, it may be the fracture of the hip due to a minor fall, or it may involve some other bone.

Osteoporosis is usually diagnosed radiologically. A good roentgenogram of the spine may be helpful, but for survey purposes, x-ray films of the hand, wrist, or jaw are more useful because in those tissues there is less variability due to soft tissue and gas overlay of the bone. In all cases the shadow of the bone shows diminished density.

Full descriptions of osteoporosis appear in the standard medical textbooks. From a nutritional point of view, there is new interest in the disease because evidence now indicates that fluoride is effective in the treatment of the disease[15,16] and may be important also in its prevention. It is known that fluoride becomes a part of the bone substance just as it does in dental enamel (Figure 9), replacing hydroxyl ions in the chemical composition of the bone and giving rise to a larger bone crystal that may be less liable to resorption.

The first evidence that fluoride intake might be an important factor in osteoporosis came from a comparison of x-ray films taken in two communities, one with low fluoride content in the water and the other with high fluoride content. Substantially more osteoporosis and decreased bone density were found in the "low-fluoride" community.[17] In another study, Bernstein et al[15] monitored osteoporosis in the populations of two North Dakota communities that were similar except for concentrations of fluoride in drinking water. As judged both by relative bone density and by the presence or absence of collapsed vertebrae, there was substantially less osteoporosis in the high-fluoride areas.

For a number of years, fluoride has been used successfully in the treatment of osteoporosis. Doses have varied from 5 to 60 mg daily, given usually as a sodium fluoride tablet. The daily dose necessary to produce remission is much larger than that which can be ingested from drinking fluoridated water. However, that does not mean that drinking fluoridated water from an early age may not help to substantially reduce osteoporosis in the elderly in the later years, although the benefit remains to be proved.

There was a widely held belief that calcium deficiencies in the diets of the elderly were important in the causation of osteoporosis. That belief is now disputed[18] because there are no good studies to substantiate such a claim. Calcium has not been effective in treatment of the disease, and there is no sound epidemiological evidence to show that osteoporosis is more prevalent where diets are commonly calcium deficient. In fact, osteoporosis has been shown to be an important problem in the United States, Great Britain, and Scandinavia—three areas where calcium intakes tend to be high.

NUTRITION AND CANCER

The death rates for many site-specific carcinomas vary widely among the world population groups for which reliable statistics are available. Furthermore, the frequencies of various site-specific carcinomas show definite time-related trends within populations. For example, the frequency of stomach cancer has decreased dramatically over the past 40 years in the United States, whereas the frequency of lung cancer has increased correspondingly.

Epidemiologic studies have shown that migrating populations eventually demonstrate cancer-related morbidity and mortality that are typical of the indigenous populations whose environments they share—and perhaps quite different from those of their native country. About 80% of cancers are "environmentally determined," but only in the specific cases of tobacco, alcohol, ionizing radiation, and certain occupation-linked cancers have specific factors been proved.

Just as diet has been epidemiologically identified as an important determinant of atherosclerosis, there is much suggestive evidence relating diet to cancer.[19] That hypothesis is strongly supported by studies with rodents in which chemical carcinogenesis was affected by diet. Proof of causality in human beings is not yet available except for a few special cases in which dietary contaminants have been strongly linked to cancer (aflatoxins to liver cancer in some tropical countries, for example). In this section, we will not consider the possible role of food contaminants or additives in carcinogenesis but will focus rather on the role of natural products.

Total calories: In human beings, obesity is associated with a modestly increased risk of developing cancer, particularly endometrial and breast cancer in females. The life span of laboratory animals is greatly prolonged by dietary restriction (ie, leanness) and shortened by obesity; interestingly, the incidence of both spontaneous and chemically induced cancers is also affected – lean animals develop fewer.

A comparable and possibly related phenomenon is that of the very low prevalence of (human) colon, breast, endometrial, and prostatic cancer in developing countries – where overeating is not a common nutritional problem.

Fats: The worldwide epidemiology of colon and breast cancers is similar to that of atherosclerosis: in human beings there is a reasonably strong correlation between intake of animal fats and risk of disease. High concentrations of dietary fats are associated with increased susceptibility to chemically induced mammary and colon cancers in laboratory animals as well. Possibly, a dietary effect on prolactin or estrogen concentrations is related to breast cancer, and perhaps the bacterial degradation products of bile acids (the concentrations of which are increased by high-fat, high-cholesterol diets) yield metabolites that could induce cancer of the colon. Diets in developing countries (in which the rates of colon cancer are generally low) are typically high in fiber content. Thus, fiber, which increases stool bulk and shortens the time that food residues are in the colon, may be a protective factor.

Vitamin A: Deficiency of vitamin A predisposes laboratory animals to the entire spectrum of chemically induced epithelial neoplasms. Conversely, certain newly synthesized and relatively nontoxic analogs of vitamin A evidently increase resistance to those neoplasms in animals. Whether vitamin A plays a role in human cancer is not known.

Benzyl isothiocyanate, the additives BHA and BHT, and the natural substances indoles and flavones have been identified as dietary inducers of the mixed-function oxidase systems, which are responsible for both the activation and the detoxification of chemical carcinogens. The prevalence of cancer in animals is decreased by the dietary inducers, the natural forms of which are found in grasses and many leafy green vegetables. BHA and BHT, synthetic antioxidants widely used as preservatives for fat-containing foods, may also have an anticarcinogenic effect.

Vegetarian diets may be beneficial in reducing the prevalence of cancer in human beings, as evidenced by preliminary analysis of a study concerning cancer rates in Seventh-Day Adventists, a religious denomination that advocates vegetarian diets (but also, it should be noted, abstinence from smoking, alcohol, and caffeine). Mortality from the commonest carcinomas among Seventh-Day Adventists is only 50% to 60% of that reported for the general population in the United States.

IRON-DEFICIENCY ANEMIA

Iron deficiency is one of the most common nutritional deficiencies in the United States. It occurs most frequently in infants beyond six months of age, in adolescent girls, and in women of childbearing age.

There are difficulties in defining iron deficiency. The sequence of events during iron depletion is believed to be (a) a loss of iron stores (which may be estimated by staining marrow smears for iron and by determining serum ferritin and erythrocyte protoporphyrin concentrations), (b) a decrease in plasma iron concentrations ($50 \mu g/dl$ is normal) with an increase in iron-binding capacity of plasma (normally over 10% saturation), and (c) the development of anemia (with characteristic low hemoglobin and hematocrit values), which in severe iron deficiency is usually a hypochromic microcytic anemia. The frequency with which iron deficiency is encountered will depend upon the criteria used for diagnosis. The commonly used measurements of hemoglobin and hematocrit undoubtedly underestimate the extent of iron depletion.[20]

Iron absorption is influenced by many factors. In general, only about 10% of dietary iron is believed to be absorbed. The adult male loses only about 0.5 to 1.0 mg of iron daily; his daily requirement for iron is therefore about 10.0 mg/day. On an average monthly basis, the adult premenopausal woman loses about twice that amount. Similarly, iron is lost during childbirth and in lactation; additional dietary iron is needed by pregnant women and growing children.

The availability of iron in foods varies greatly. In general, heme iron is well absorbed from foods of animal origin (meat, poultry, and fish), but the iron present in vegetable products, including cereals such as wheat, corn, and rice, is poorly absorbed. These differences may be modified by a mixture of foods consumed together. It is well known that phytates and phosphates, present in cereal grains, inhibit iron absorption. On the other hand, protein and ascorbic acid (vitamin C) enhance iron absorption. Recent research has shown that ascorbic acid mixed with table salt and added to cereals will increase the absorption of intrinsic iron in cereals twofold to fourfold.[21] The consumption of vitamin-C-rich foods such as fresh fruits and vegetables with a meal may therefore promote iron absorption. Egg yolk impairs the absorption of iron, even though eggs are one of the better sources of food iron.

In the adult, iron deficiency is frequently associated with blood loss. In many parts of the world, excessive blood loss is associated with hookworm infestation, which can lead to severe iron-deficiency anemia. Increased requirements for iron are also associated with growth, iron being required for all cells and particularly for the increase in blood volume. Iron deficiency is frequently encountered in infants, especially in those born to anemic mothers. The normal infant is born with iron stores, but milk is a very poor source of iron. Supplemental iron-rich foods or formulas are therefore indicated to prevent anemia in the latter part of infancy or early childhood. Anemia and iron depletion is common in adolescent girls, who bear the combined stress of growth and menstruation. Pregnancy also imposes the stress of fetal growth combined with an expansion of the blood volume. Women with poor dietary habits often enter pregnancy with reduced iron stores.

Variations in iron requirements and in iron utilization make it difficult to estimate the iron requirement of any individual. The Recommended Dietary Allowances (RDA) are set on the high side so that the needs of the majority will be met. The (1974) RDA for women are higher than previously recommended allowances and will probably not be met by the usual diets in the United States. The questions are therefore posed: Should the usual diet contain enough iron to meet the needs of persons with high iron requirements? If so, how can that be accomplished? Most bread and flour in the United States are fortified with iron, and the quantity of iron could be increased. However, women and girls do not ordinarily consume large amounts of bread. Thus, foods other than bread should be considered for iron fortification.

Anemia is known to cause various symptoms such as tiredness, weakness, and dyspnea on exertion; when severe, anemia may lead to tachycardia, palpitations, and edema. Severe anemia in pregnant women increases maternal morbidity and mortality and confers a higher risk for the fetus. A number of studies have shown that physical work capacity is reduced in persons with low hemoglobin concentrations. Increasing evidence suggests that iron deficiency may play a role in limiting one's ability to resist infection. For example, concentrations of the cytoplasmic enzyme myeloperoxidase in granulocytes may be decreased in persons with iron deficiency, decreasing the cells' ability to fight bacterial infections. Iron deficiency may also impair humoral antibody response.

In the United States, control of iron deficiency is complicated by the fact that total food intake becomes smaller as the population becomes more sedentary and as many girls and women are concerned about obesity. When the total caloric intake is low and when approximately 40% of the calories are supplied as fat and 15% to 20% as sugar, there is little room in the diet for iron-containing foods. Improved manufacturing methods, the use of stainless steel and aluminum (rather than cast iron) utensils, and emphasis on cleanliness have lowered the total iron intake. Although iron toxicity (hemosiderosis and hemochromatosis) exists, it is rare and probably hereditary; its prevalence is unlikely to be increased by more-adequate fortification of foods with iron. In our opinion, it is indeed unfortunate that the Commissioner of the FDA overruled a previous decision of the FDA to increase substantially the amount of iron fortification of enriched flour and bread.

PROTEIN-CALORIE MALNUTRITION IN YOUNG CHILDREN

Protein-calorie malnutrition in young children constitutes the most important and widespread nutritional problem in the world today. The two main clinical syndromes are kwashiorkor and nutritional marasmus. In kwashiorkor the principal deficiency is of protein, whereas in marasmus there is an overall deficit in food intake resulting in insufficient calories and protein. From the clinical point of view, there are many intermediate cases that are difficult to fit into either category; they show some of the symptoms and signs of both conditions.

It should be recalled that these clinical entities constitute only the relatively small exposed part of the enormous iceberg of protein-calorie malnutrition. For every frank case of serious clinical protein-calorie deficiency disease, there are perhaps 99 children who are receiving an inadequate diet, who are grown poorly, and who are prone to infections. Those 99 children have mild or subclinical cases of protein-calorie malnutrition, and typically they remain "submerged" in the population of children. They are liable to be precipitated into one of these clinical states by any of a variety of causes.

Over the past two decades, kwashiorkor has been recognized and studied in many parts of the world and is now accepted as one disease with a few local variations. During this

Figure 10. Clinical features of kwashiorkor and marasmus compared.[22]

Clinical Feature	Kwashiorkor	Marasmus
Growth failure	Present	Present
Edema	Present	Absent
Mental changes	Present	Uncommon
Hepatomegaly	Common	Uncommon
Hair changes	Common	Uncommon
Dermatosis (flaky paint)	Fairly common	Absent
Anemia	Very common	Common
Subcutaneous fat	Reduced but present	Absent
Appetite	Poor	Good

period, the emphasis has been on protein deficiency, and a worldwide effort has been made to increase the quantity and quality of protein available to children. More recently, attention has turned to the equal importance of a shortage of calories as part of an overall deficiency of food in the diets of young children.

Kwashiorkor and nutritional marasmus can be regarded as the two extremes of protein-calorie malnutrition of young children. However, very many cases of protein-calorie malnutrition are intermediate, and this has given rise to such names as "marasmic kwashiorkor" to describe cases in which kwashiorkor is superimposed on marasmus. Separate descriptions are given kwashiorkor and nutritional marasmus, but the clinicians must expect many cases to be intermediate between the two extremes (Figure 10).

Kwashiorkor

Etiology and epidemiology: Kwashiorkor occurs mainly in children 1 to 3 years of age. It is common in many developing countries of Asia, Africa, and Latin America, but has been reported also in Europe and the United States, where it is associated with poverty.

The disease occurs in children whose diet is grossly deficient in protein. Often the food that the child is receiving is of a type that contains mostly carbohydrate and little protein. In many parts of the world, kwashiorkor is a disease of the weaning period when the child is taken from the breast and given a diet that is primarily starch. An adequate intake of breast milk will provide a satisfactory diet for the first four to six months of an infant's life. After that, chiefly because of reduced quantities, breast milk provides merely a useful protein-rich dietary supplement to whatever other food the child is receiving.

Important factors often implicated in the complex etiology of kwashiorkor are:

a The rapid growth and relatively high protein requirements of the rapidly growing young child

b A protein-poor, staple food for the child, eg, manioc, bananas, sugar

c Poor infant-feeding practices

d A lack of protein-rich foods, both animal (eg, meat, milk, fish, eggs) and vegetable (eg, beans, peanuts)

e Poor distribution of available food in the family (eg, the adults and older children often get the major share of protein-rich foods such as meat)

Figure 11. Kwashiorkor in an African child showing edema and dermatosis.

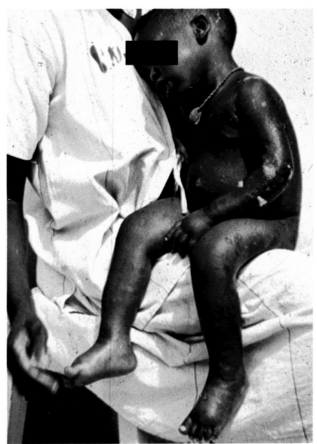

f Seasonal food shortages

g Poverty and its attendant ills

h Cultural dietary practices, including food taboos, may preclude the child's consumption of certain available and nutritionally desirable foods

i Infections such as diarrhea, measles, whooping cough

j Ignorance or lack of knowledge on the part of parents or guardians concerning what foods are needed in the child's diet

k Psychological factors that may affect the appetite of the child

The disease: Below are the main features of kwashiorkor:

a *Growth failure* is always present. If the child's age is known he will be found to be shorter and, except in cases with gross edema, lighter than normal.

b *Wasting* is always a feature, but it may be masked by edema. The wasting is often evident in the muscles of the arms and legs.

c *Edema* always occurs and is a most important feature of the disease (Figure 11). It may affect any part of the body. In an ambulant child, edema usually starts as a slight swelling of the feet and often spreads up the legs. Later the hands, scrotum, and face may all be affected.

d *Mental changes* are invariably present. The child is usually apathetic and uninterested in his surroundings. At the same time he is miserable and irritable when being moved or disturbed. He is unsmiling and his behavioral development is retarded.

e *Hair changes* are common. The hair often shows changes in texture, in color, in strength, and in ease of pluckability. The tight curl of African or Afro-American hair is often lost and the hair becomes silkier and loses its lustre. Black hair becomes brown or reddish brown. In Latin America, parallel strips of discolored hair have been labeled the "flag sign."

f *Skin changes* are not invariable, but if present may be very characteristic (Figure 12). The skin, especially of the face, may show depigmentation. In some cases dermatosis develops, especially in areas of friction such as the groins and behind the knees. Darkly pigmented patches appear and may desquamate like old blistered paint – a phenomenon that has given rise to the term "flaky-paint dermatosis." Beneath the flakes are atrophic areas that may resemble a healing burn.

g *Diarrhea* is common. Stools are frequently loose and contain undigested particles of food. Sometimes they are offensive, watery, and blood stained.

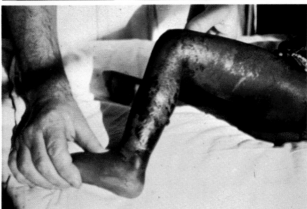

Figure 12. Kwashiorkor – skin lesions.

Figure 13. Fatty infiltration of the liver in kwashiorkor.

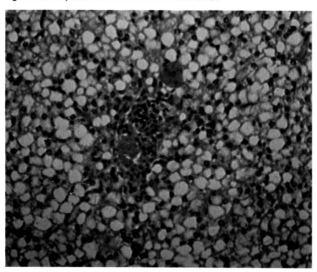

h *Anemia* to some degree is common in most cases of kwashiorkor. This is due in part to a lack of protein to synthesize blood cells but is frequently complicated by anemia resulting in iron deficiency, hookworm infestation, malaria, etc.

i *Hepatomegaly* is due to fatty infiltration of the liver, which is always found post mortem in kwashiorkor (Figure 13).

j *Signs of other deficiencies* are usual. There is usually some subcutaneous fat in persons with kwashiorkor; in marasmus there is usually none or very little. The degree of fat deficiency gives an indication of the degree of calorie deficiency. Lesions of the lips and mouth characteristic of vitamin B deficiencies may be seen, and xerosis or xerophthalmia due to vitamin A deficiency may sometimes be present.

Laboratory findings: In kwashiorkor the total serum protein concentration is reduced, with the serum albumin content reduced more than the globulin content. Serum amylase and pancreatic enzyme concentrations are also reduced as is the ratio of essential to nonessential amino acids. Serum transferrin levels are also low, and the extent of the reduction gives a good index of the severity of the disease. Liver biopsy reveals fatty infiltration, but despite the presence of edema, there is no albumin in the urine.

Treatment: All patients with severe kwashiorkor should, if possible, be admitted to a hospital for treatment. Severity is judged by the degree of edema; the extent of dermatosis; the hemoglobin level; the severity of diarrhea, vomiting, and dehydration; the willingness of the child to feed; but above all by the general clinical condition of the patient.

Dried skimmed milk is a most satisfactory basis for treatment, but other protein-rich foods are effective. A mixture of dried skimmed milk, vegetable oil, and casein is ideal; if necessary the child can be given the mixture through an intragastric tube. The milk should provide about 120 calories and 7 gm of protein per kg of body weight per day.

If diarrhea is severe, approximately 0.5 gm potassium chloride in water should be given three times a day.

Antibiotics should be given to combat infection. In malarial areas, chloroquine or some other antimalarial drug is also desirable.

When shock, severe anemia, or dehydration occurs, appropriate supportive measures are indicated. In cases of shock or if the anemia is severe, a blood transfusion might prove life-saving. Anemia of a moderate nature can be treated with orally or parenterally administered iron.

Severe dehydration calls for the intravenous administration of electrolyte solutions.

Vitamins should be given for vitamin deficiencies; it is especially important to treat any evidence of eye changes caused by vitamin A deficiency.

Severe cases of kwashiorkor can be expected to respond quite rapidly to the above regimen. The diarrhea and gastrointestinal symptoms subside, diuresis occurs with rapid reduction of edema, and, as the anorexia disappears, the mood of the child begins to change – a smile may be a good prognostic sign.

At this stage the treatment can be modified and will be similar for mild cases not requiring hospitalization – consisting of a more-varied diet rich in protein. The mother's cooperation in the dietary regimen is important and should form an integral part of therapy so as to expand her nutritional education.

Nutritional Marasmus

Etiology and epidemiology: Nutritional marasmus is common in nearly all developing countries and, in contrast to kwashiorkor, is more common among children younger than 1 year, although it is not restricted to this age group. The disease is a form of starvation and therefore the underlying causes are numerous but all involve serious lack of food (Figure 14). In the United States, nutritional marasmus is occasionally seen in grossly neglected children but may also occur secondary to such diseases as cystic fibrosis, celiac disease, or overwhelming infections.

A common cause of nutritional marasmus among peoples of developing countries is early cessation of breast feeding. This may be due to death of the mother, failure of lactation, separation of the infant from the mother, or most commonly the mother's desire to feed her infant from the bottle rather than the breast. In this latter event she may be influenced by advertisements and the impact of alien cultures into believing that bottle feeding is superior or more sophisticated. Early cessation of breast feeding does not of course necessarily lead to marasmus. However, a large proportion of people in developing countries do not have sufficient income to purchase enough milk formula to feed a baby properly. As a result, the tendency is to overdilute the mixture with water, which then fails to provide adequate calories. Similarly, few in these countries have a safe water supply or items in their homes with which to simplify the sterile preparation of bottles of formula for an infant. Combined with a lack of knowledge concerning hygiene, those problems commonly lead to the development of gastrointestinal infection, which starts the vicious circle leading to marasmus.

Other common causes of marasmus are prematurity and gastrointestinal diseases such as diarrhea or malabsorption. Many of the factors that cause kwashiorkor may also be involved.

The disease: Following are the main features of nutritional marasmus:

a *Growth failure* is clearly evident in all cases. If the age of the child is known, the weight will be seen to be extremely low by normal standards, and the height will also usually be below normal. In severe cases the wasting of flesh is obvious. The ribs are prominent, the face has a characteristic monkey-like appearance, the limbs are very thin, but the abdomen may be protuberant. In general, the child looks like the starved person he is.

b *Wasting* of muscles is extreme. There is little if any subcutaneous fat remaining. The skin hangs in wrinkles, especially around the buttocks and thighs.

c *The appetite* is good. Whereas the child with kwashiorkor has anorexia, the child with marasmus frequently has a good appetite. In fact, like any starving creature, he may be ravenous, often sucking his hands and clothing.

d *The mental state* appears to be unaffected. Most children with marasmus appear bright eyed and alert. They are not

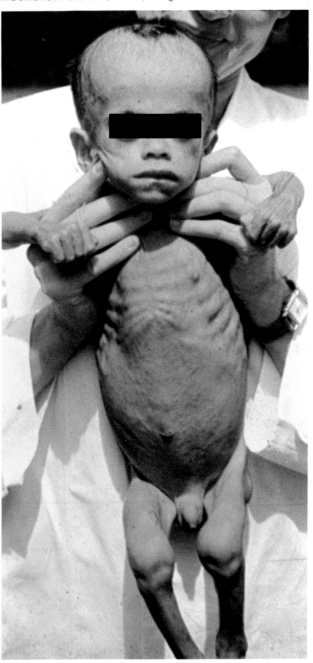

Figure 14. Nutritional marasmus, showing extreme wasting in a child from Rotterdam, Holland, during World War II.

usually disinterested or irritable, as are children with kwashiorkor.

e *Anemia* is usually present.

f *Diarrhea* is common, but is not a constant feature.

An advanced case of nutritional marasmus presents an unmistakable picture. The infant is appallingly thin but, in contrast to the rest of the body, the belly may be protuberant. The disease, unlike kwashiorkor, does not lead to edema or flaky-paint dermatosis. Hair changes similar to those seen in kwashiorkor can occur but are less common. Signs of vitamin deficiency, especially of vitamin A, may accompany marasmus.

Laboratory findings: Serum protein concentrations may be reduced, but less so than in kwashiorkor.

The hydroxyproline-creatinine index is low,[23] but the ratio of essential to nonessential amino acids is less altered than in kwashiorkor.

The liver is not infiltrated with fat.

Treatment: Treatment is similar to that described for kwashiorkor, but an adequate intake of calories and protein is mandatory to allow for weight gain and growth. Therefore, if dried skimmed milk is used as the basis for treatment, vegetable oil should be added to provide calories.

Anemia, infections, diarrhea, and dehydration should be treated as described for kwashiorkor. In general, response to treatment in severe nutritional marasmus is slow, and prolonged hospitalization is often necessary.

It is particularly important to ensure that the child is not discharged from treatment only to return to the very set of circumstances that led to the disease. Steps must be taken to ensure that an adequate diet is provided for the child after he leaves the hospital.

Mild to Moderate Protein-Calorie Malnutrition

Although detailed descriptions of kwashiorkor and nutritional marasmus have been given, one should note that these are extreme clinical conditions in the wide spectrum that constitutes protein-calorie malnutrition. In practice, many intermediate forms will be encountered. More important, however, is the fact that for every clinical case of each of these diseases there are hundreds of children who have mild or moderate forms of protein-calorie malnutrition. From a public health point of view, it is desirable to try to detect these mild cases and in some way prevent them from becoming severe.

The best means of detecting mild degrees of protein-calorie malnutrition is to follow the growth and development of young children. A child who fails to grow normally is a candidate for severe protein-calorie malnutrition, and the one factor that most frequently leads to a deterioration of nutritional status is an infectious disease.

Ideally, heights, weights, and other measures of development should be followed secularly in all children at risk. If this is not possible, then growth failure, as indicated by low height or weight for age, forms a useful guide. There are at present no sufficiently developed biochemical tests to provide a better means of detecting early protein-calorie malnutrition than the measurement of height and weight.

A grading of malnutrition on the basis of weight-for-age is widely used in developing countries. This is the Gomez classification[24]:

Grade I Malnutrition –
75% to 90% of expected weight-for-age
Grade II Malnutrition –
60% to 75% of expected weight-for-age
Grade III Malnutrition –
less than 60% of expected weight-for-age

A child can of course lose weight very rapidly because of illness or gross dietary deficiencies. In contrast, height once acquired cannot be lost except in aging adulthood. Height deficits therefore provide a better indication of chronic malnutrition. However, height expressed as a percentage of normal height gives a false picture in that it indicates smaller deficits than does weight. It is better to state height-age as a percentage of actual age.[25] For example, if the standard age for reaching 84 cm in height is 24 months, then a child who is 84 cm at age 36 months is 66% of his height-age.

Other anthropometric measures that have practical value include head circumference, chest circumference, upper-arm circumference, and skinfold thickness.[26]

Malnutrition and subsequent development: There is good scientific evidence to show that children who have suffered from protein-calorie malnutrition early in life have some permanent stunting of physical growth. Therefore, if the malnutrition has been prolonged, serious dwarfing may result.

There is some evidence to suggest that protein-calorie malnutrition early in life may also result in failure of the child to reach his full potential of intellectual and psychological development.[27] In experimental animals it has been shown that behavioral abnormalities follow early malnutrition.

By relating DNA to cell numbers, it has also been found that baby rats malnourished during the suckling period subsequently have reduced numbers of brain cells.[28]

A few studies have indicated that children who have had malnutrition early in life subsequently perform less well on a variety of mental tests than do children of the same age who have not had malnutrition. There are indications that malnourished children may never catch up to the other children in intelligence.[29] Some studies have also shown that malnourished children also have reduced head circumference, a measure that may provide an indication of brain size.[30]

Research on the relationship of malnutrition to behavioral development is relatively recent. Therefore, although early protein-calorie malnutrition is definitely associated with subsequent poor intellectual performance, the relationship has not been proved to be one of cause and effect. Quite possibly, some genetic and other environmental factors that influence intellectual development of children may also be important in the etiology of malnutrition. Therefore, factors such as poverty, ignorant or illiterate parents, overcrowding, a high prevalence of infectious disease, poor learning opportunities, and several others may be causes both of malnutrition and of poor psychological development in children.

Nutrition and Infection

In recent years, the importance of the synergism of infection and dietary deficiencies in the causation of severe protein-calorie malnutrition has been realized.[31, 32] The corollary is equally true: namely, that malnutrition is largely responsible for the increased severity and many of the devastating effects of infectious disease in malnourished children. Gastroenteritis, measles, and other infections may frequently precipitate clinical malnutrition in a child. Similarly, some diseases (such as measles) that are associated with very low mortality in the well-nourished often result in high mortality among populations in which malnutrition is prevalent.

Diarrheal disease in children who are being weaned from the breast is extremely common in developing countries and has been termed "weaning diarrhea." The disorder is now commonly known to be a precipitating cause of malnutrition. It is also now clear that malnourished children more frequently develop diarrhea than do the well-nourished and that frequently the diarrhea may be due to malnutrition and not to a pathogenic organism.

NUTRITION IN PREGNANCY AND DURING LACTATION[33]

During gestation, the fetus derives all calories and nutrients from the maternal circulation. The mother's circulation, in turn, is supplied from her storage depots and from her diet, which must also satisfy her own requirements. A normal, well-fed woman has significant reserves of protein in her muscles, energy in her adipose tissue, and calcium in her skeleton, as well as other essential nutrients that can be called upon to support fetal growth and development.

The child's birth weight – the most widely used indicator of pregnancy outcome – is influenced by maternal height and weight before pregnancy (which reflect maternal reserves) as well as by maternal weight gain during pregnancy (which is a function of diet and physical activity). Maternal age and the interval between pregnancies have also been shown to influence birth weight; these relationships may also be mediated by nutrition. Closely spaced pregnancies tend to deplete maternal reserves; teenage mothers, who are themselves still in the process of growing, have additional nutritional requirements, and frequently, insufficient and poorly balanced diets.

The nutritional status of the mother during her own childhood also influences birth weight and obstetrical risk. Tall women who have fully realized their own growth potential have favorable pelvic outlets, fewer obstetrical complications, and give birth to well-developed babies. Short women who were stunted during their own childhood or affected with rickets have flattened pelvic outlets and, consequently, a relatively high incidence of cephalopelvic disproportion. Their children are likely to be underweight at birth (less than 2500 gm).

In optimal nutritional circumstances, women gain on the average of 12.5 kg during pregnancy. Besides formation of new fetal and placental tissue and growth of the uterus and breasts, there is a significant increment of maternal adipose tissue stores, which help support lactation. The energy costs of pregnancy, including calories present as maternal reserves at the time of birth, are estimated to be close to 80,000 Calories. Approximately half of this requirement is usually met by increments in dietary intake; the other half is met by reduction in customary physical activity. To achieve the normal 12.5 kg maternal weight gain that is associated with optimal birth weight and minimum neonatal mortality, maternal dietary intake must be increased. The Recommended Dietary Allowances (Table I, page 14) summarize the increments required to ensure optimal fetal development and prevention of maternal depletion. These recommendations can be easily met with a well-balanced diet that includes one quart of milk per day to compensate for, particularly, increased calcium needs. Some obstetricians recommend dietary supplementation with iron and folic acid to prevent the maternal deficits that may occur physiologically. Other obstetricians prescribe the supplements only when iron deficiency or megaloblastic anemia is detected.

Protein-Calorie Malnutrition (PCM) During Pregnancy

On a worldwide basis, deficiency in energy and protein intake is by far the most important nutritional disorder during pregnancy. Like PCM in childhood, the problem is associated with poverty and unsanitary environments. The latter are thought to increase the risk of intrauterine infection. It follows that the effects of PCM during pregnancy are a function of both the mother's nutritional status before pregnancy and the degree of dietary insufficiency during pregnancy. During the World War II siege of Leningrad, most of the city's women were limited to diets that provided less than 1000 Calories and 30 gm of low-quality protein daily. Superimposed on prior maternal malnourishment and increased work loads, those extreme conditions had profound effects on maternal and fetal health and on reproductive competence. Amenorrhea and consequent reduced fertility became prevalent. The number of stillbirths doubled, and the incidence of low birth weight increased dramatically – as did perinatal mortality. Severe nutritional deprivation was also prevalent in Holland near the end of World War II, but there, where women were previously well nourished, reduction in birth weight and other effects were much less severe.

The incidence of low birth weight (less than 2500 gm) varies with socioeconomic class. In developing countries, the association is presumably mediated by maternal nutritional status before pregnancy and during gestation. Diminished birth weight is, in turn, associated with high neonatal mortality, neurological disorders, and substandard cognitive development and school performance. Whether or not this relationship is a causal one remains to be established, since the incidence of low birth weight co-varies with other detrimental characteristics of impoverished environments that may themselves affect health and child development. Two recent observations suggest, however, that low birth weight

itself is the cause of high neonatal mortality: (1) The birth-weight-specific neonatal death rate is similar throughout the various socioeconomic classes, and (2) perinatal mortality has been reduced by nutritional supplementation during the last trimester of pregnancy.

These data as well as results of experiments with both animals and humans show permanent reduction in brain cellularity and protein content as a result of extreme dietary restrictions during pregnancy and immediately following birth (ie, during the critical period of rapid brain growth). Such studies suggest that priority should be given to the prevention of PCM among pregnant women in all areas of the world.

Restriction of weight gain during pregnancy to prevent obesity is still practiced in affluent societies. Clearly, weight-gain restriction for normal-weight women cannot be justified. More information is needed to guide clinical practice on the effects of moderate weight-gain restriction among obese pregnant women. In any case, careful attention must be paid to providing a varied and complete diet as well as iron and vitamin supplements when needed during this critical stage of the life cycle.

Lactation

Mother's milk is the best source of nourishment for the infant. This is particularly true in developing countries and underprivileged areas where formula feeding is associated with a dual danger: contamination of the water used in preparation of the formula, and insufficient funds to purchase enough formula to satisfy the baby's nutritional requirements.

Per dl, human milk supplies 70 Calories, 1.2 gm of protein, 30 mg of calcium, and other nutrients. Maternal production of 8 to 9 dl of milk per day, taking into consideration the efficiency of conversion, requires 800 Calories, 10 gm of protein, and 275 mg of calcium. The recommended increments in dietary allowances are 500 Calories, 20 gm protein, and 400 mg of calcium per day. The caloric allowance takes into consideration the adipose tissue stores accumulated during pregnancy, approximately 25,000 Calories, which can be tapped at the rate of 300 Calories per day for about three months. If lactation continues beyond that time, maternal calorie intake may need to be increased if weight loss is to be avoided. Since production of milk with appropriate protein and calcium content must be maintained in spite of insufficient dietary intake, it is evident that maternal stores may be depleted by an insufficient diet during lactation. If such depletion is superimposed on closely spaced pregnancies, maternal undernourishment will lead to low birth weight and, consequently, to high rates of neonatal mortality and morbidity. Lactating women therefore deserve high priority in the planning of nutritional policy and clinical services.

XEROPHTHALMIA AND VITAMIN A DEFICIENCY

Xerophthalmia, which is the clinical manifestation of vitamin A deficiency, is quite rare in the United States but is a common cause of blindness in some parts of the world, particularly in Asia. It is caused by a diet deficient in vitamin A and its precursor, carotene. The disease occurs most commonly in young children and is often associated with protein-calorie malnutrition.

The Disease

An early sign of vitamin A deficiency is night blindness (the inability to see well in dim light), which may be difficult to detect objectively, especially in young children (Figure 15). Although vitamin A deficiency may also cause follicular hyperkeratosis of the skin, the characteristic lesions of the disease are seen in the eye (Figures 16, 17, and 18). Xerophthalmia usually begins with a drying of the conjunctiva, which then loses its shining luster. This condition of conjunctival xerosis may be accompanied by thickening, wrinkling, or pigmentation of the conjunctiva. Another common lesion that may or may not be present is Bitot spots — usually small, foamy, oval or triangular plaques situated on the bulbar conjunctiva. The spots are nearly always bilateral, temporally situated, and are sometimes associated with conjunctival xerosis.

The drying of the eye may then spread to the cornea, which develops a lusterless and rough appearance termed *corneal xerosis*. If the disease progresses, corneal ulceration may develop with loss of corneal substance. At this stage, there are often no signs or only mild signs of reaction or redness due to inflammation. If the condition is not treated, a softening necrosis ensues, leading to deformation and later to destruction of the eyeball. The process, known as keratomalacia, is often rapid — the cornea "melts" away, often with loss of vitreous fluid and sometimes with extrusion of the lens. The patient with keratomalacia is nearly always seriously ill, and blindness is a common result in those who survive.

If treatment is begun at the stage of corneal ulceration, the

Vitamin A deficiency — Night blindness is a practical and early diagnostic sign of vitamin A deficiency. The loss of visual acuity in dim light following exposure to bright light is illustrated.

Figure 15A. Both the normal person and the vitamin A-deficient patient see the headlights of an approaching car, as shown.

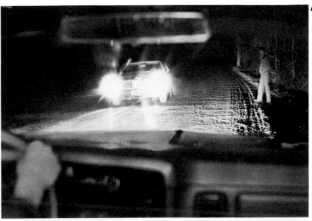

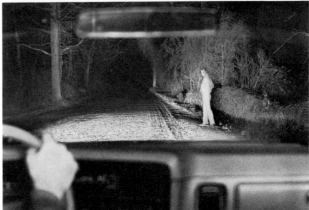

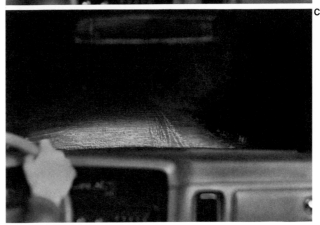

Figure 15B. After the car has passed, the normal person sees a wide stretch of road.

Figure 15C. The vitamin A-deficient patient can barely see a few feet ahead and cannot see the pedestrian at all.

36

Figure 16. Xerophthalmia.

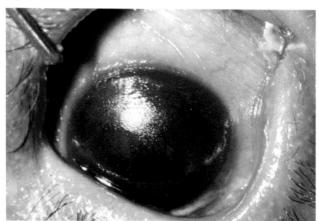

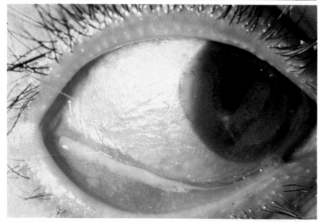

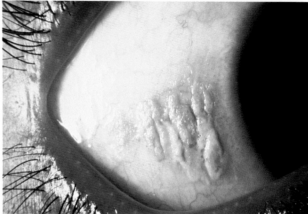

Figure 17. Generalized xerophthalmia.

Figure 18. "Cheesy" xerophthalmia.

ulcer may heal and leave only opaque corneal scars, which will then be the permanent sequelae of the disease. Clinical xerophthalmia is now classified[34] as follows:

Classification	Primary Signs
X1A	Conjunctival xerosis
X1B	Bitot spots, with conjunctival xerosis
X2	Corneal xerosis
X3A	Corneal ulceration with xerosis
X3B	Keratomalacia

Classification	Secondary Signs
XN	Night blindness
XF	Xerophthalmia fundus
XS	Corneal scars

In human beings, biochemical changes precede the development of eye lesions. Serum concentrations of vitamin A in normally nourished persons are often about 40 μg/dl. Serum concentrations of vitamin A are usually classified as:

High	= more than 50 μg/dl
Normal	= 20 to 50 μg/dl
Low	= 10 to 20 μg/dl
Deficient	= less than 10 μg/dl

Vitamin A is stored in the liver, so hepatic concentrations of vitamin A are invariably very low in patients with vitamin A deficiency (but are difficult to measure in the living subject, especially under field conditions). Vitamin A is transported by retinol-binding protein (RBP), concentrations of which are also low in persons with vitamin A deficiency.[35]

Treatment
Severe cases of xerophthalmia should be treated as medical emergencies, because both the sight and life of affected children are at stake. The recommended treatment is:
a An intramuscular injection of 100,000 IU of a water-miscible vitamin A preparation immediately upon admission to the hospital.
b Unless contraindicated by vomiting or nausea, an oral dose of 100,000 IU vitamin A (in combination with vitamin E) in oily solution on the day after admission.
c A second oral dose of the same preparation just before discharge. For children less than one year old, the dose

is 100,000 IU; for those older than one year, the dose is 200,000 IU.

Oily solutions of vitamin A are no longer administered by intramuscular injection, because the vitamin is liberated slowly, if at all, from the injection site. The preferred, active form of vitamin A is retinol palmitate in a water-miscible preparation.

Response to treatment is often dramatic, and any failure to respond may indicate misdiagnosis. Underlying conditions such as protein-calorie malnutrition, gastroenteritis, dehydration, and infections must be treated appropriately and concurrently.

Prevention and Control

The prevention of xerophthalmia in children at risk depends on a diet rich in carotene or vitamin A and on the control of associated diseases such as protein-calorie malnutrition, measles, and diarrhea. As a long-term public health measure, prevention and control may require alleviating poverty, improving living standards, and increasing the production of appropriate foods. In the meantime, certain other measures may be effective and feasible:

a *Fortification of suitable foods with appropriate doses of vitamin A.* In the United States, several common foods are fortified with vitamin A. In developing countries, a number of foods are being fortified especially to control xerophthalmia. These include sugar in Central America, tea in India, and monosodium glutamate (MSG) in the Philippines.

b *Periodic massive-dose programs.* Vitamin A, being a fat-soluble vitamin, is stored in the liver. In a number of countries, susceptible children are periodically given massive doses of vitamin A to prevent xerophthalmia. Typically, 200,000 IU of vitamin A in oil with vitamin E is given orally at six-month intervals. Recent evidence, however, suggests that serum concentrations of vitamin A decline to their original levels by the end of six months. The dose should therefore be given every four months (or half that dose – 100,000 IU – every two months). The problem with massive dosing is the difficulty in having an appropriate delivery system that regularly reaches susceptible children.

By far the best practical report on xerophthalmia is A. Somer's *Field Guide to the Detection and Control of Xerophthalmia*, published by the World Health Organization. The book is available from Helen Keller International, 22 West 17th Street, New York, New York 10011.

THIAMIN DEFICIENCY SYNDROMES, INCLUDING BERIBERI AND WERNICKE-KORSAKOFF SYNDROME

Beriberi: The Disease

Beriberi is caused by a deficiency of the B vitamin thiamin, also known as B_1, when the ratio of its intake to the number of calories obtained from carbohydrate is low. The disease occurs predominantly among rice-eating peoples of the world because of their use of refined or polished rice.

From a clinical viewpoint, there are various ways to classify beriberi. Here it will be grouped into three forms: (1) wet beriberi, (2) dry beriberi, and (3) infantile beriberi. These three clinical forms of the disease have many different features and yet appear to be caused by the same dietary deficiency and occur in the same endemic areas.

Early clinical features common to both wet and dry beriberi: Both wet and dry beriberi usually begin in a similar mild way. The person tires easily, his limbs feel heavy and weak, and he may get a mild degree of swelling around the ankles. There may be numbness and a feeling of "pins and needles" in the legs, as well as occasional palpitations of the heart.

Examination at this stage might reveal some reduced motor power, perhaps a slight alteration in gait, and a patchy anesthesia over the skin of the lower legs. The rice eater in the Orient or the alcoholic elsewhere will often continue his normal activities and not seek early medical advice. The condition at this stage would improve with a better diet or with thiamin administration. Left untreated, the condition might remain almost static for months but at an early stage might progress to either clinical wet or dry beriberi.

Wet beriberi: The name wet beriberi is used because the main feature of the disease is the accumulation of fluid in the legs and often in the scrotum, face, and trunk (Figure 19). The patient frequently develops cardiac palpitations, chest pain, and later, dyspnea. The pulse is rapid and often irregular. The neck veins are distended with visible pulsations, and the heart becomes enlarged. The volume of urine tends to be diminished but, despite the edema, contains no albumin. This latter is an important diagnostic feature.

A patient with wet beriberi is in danger of rapid deterioration, acute circulatory failure, and death.

Dry beriberi: This is termed dry beriberi because edema is not a feature. The condition is really neuritic beriberi and is similar to peripheral neuritis due to other causes.

Anesthesia and paresthesia of the feet, followed by increased difficulty in walking, are common features. On

38

Figure 19. Edema in beriberi.

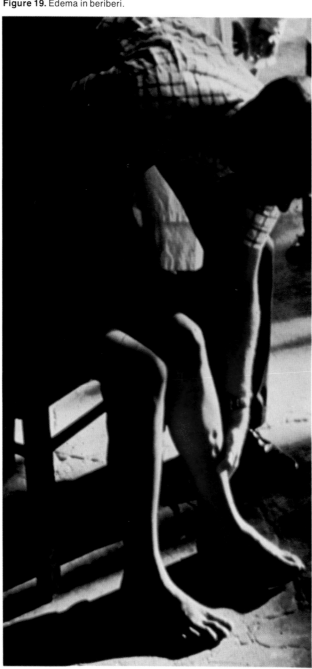

examination the patient has a peculiar ataxic gait, foot drop and wrist drop are common, there is considerable muscular wasting, there are anesthetic patches especially over the tibia, and there is tenderness of the calves and other muscles when pressure is applied. The sufferer has great difficulty in rising from the squatting position.

The disease is often chronic, and at any stage improvement may slowly occur if the subject consumes a better diet or receives treatment with thiamin. Without treatment, the disease progresses; the patient eventually becomes bedridden and, typically, dies of some chronic infection.

Infantile beriberi: This is the only important dietary deficiency disease that occurs in otherwise normal infants less than 6 months of age who are receiving adequate quantities of breast milk. It is due to inadequate thiamin in the milk of a lactating mother whose own diet is deficient in the vitamin. The mother, however, may have no overt signs of beriberi.

Infantile beriberi typically affects infants between 2 and 6 months of age. In the acute form, the infant develops dyspnea and cyanosis and, with unnerving rapidity, dies of cardiac failure. In chronic forms, the classical sign is aphonia – the infant goes through the motions of crying like a well-rehearsed mime but without emitting much of any sound. The infant is thin and wasted, diarrhea and vomiting may develop, and, because of a deficiency of calories and other nutrients, the infant becomes marasmic. Edema occasionally is seen, and convulsions may occur in the terminal stages.

Diagnosis of wet, dry, and infantile beriberi: Diagnosis may be difficult when only the early manifestations are present. A history of a diet deficient in thiamin, and relief of symptoms upon treatment with thiamin or an improved diet, will help to establish the diagnosis.

Wet beriberi must be distinguished from renal edema and congestive cardiac failure. In both latter conditions there is albuminuria; in beriberi there is not.

Measurement of blood levels of thiamin and thiamin phosphate is of limited value in diagnosis. More useful are determinations of blood lactate and blood pyruvate levels, especially if performed after dextrose administration and exercise. Urinary excretion of thiamin per gm of creatinine provides a good index of thiamin intake but is useful more for surveys than for diagnosis in the individual patient.

Treatment of wet beriberi:

a Absolute bed rest.

b Thiamin, 10 to 20 mg daily, by injection. When clinical improvement is evident, replace injections with oral thiamin, 10 mg daily.

c Full nutritious diet rich in B vitamins but low in carbohydrate.

The treatment of patients with severe wet beriberi is very gratifying, for the response is usually dramatic. Within a few days, diuresis and rapid reduction of dyspnea occur with elimination of edema.

Treatment of dry beriberi:

a Rest in bed.

b Thiamin 10 mg daily by mouth.

c Nutritious diet including B complex vitamins.

d Physiotherapy.

Improvement is often very slow.

Treatment of infantile beriberi:

a Immediate injection of thiamin 5 mg and daily injections for four days.

b Thiamin 10 mg orally twice a day to the mother if the child is being breast fed.

c Nutritious and thiamin-rich diet for both mother and child.

Thiamin Deficiency in the United States

Although classical beriberi is uncommon in the United States, thiamin deficiency is by no means a rarity. It is confined mainly to the alcoholic population. Alcoholism is an increasingly prevalent condition, and several clinical features previously believed to be due to chronic alcoholic intoxication are now known to be the result of nutritional deficiencies.

Wernicke-Korsakoff Syndrome

Wernicke's disease is characterized by eye signs (nystagmus, diplopia, paralysis of the externi recti muscles, and sometimes ophthalmoplegia), ataxia, and mental changes. Korsakoff's psychosis leads to a loss of memory of the immediate past and often an elaborate confabulation that tends to conceal this amnesia.

It is now generally agreed that any distinction between Wernicke's disease and Korsakoff's psychosis in the alcoholic patient may be artificial. Korsakoff's psychosis may be regarded as the psychotic component of Wernicke's disease.[36]

This view is supported by the fact that many patients who appear with ocular palsy, ataxia, and confusion, and who survive, later show the amnestic disorder of Korsakoff's psychosis. Similarly, patients with Korsakoff's psychosis who are in psychiatric institutions often show the stigmata of Wernicke's disease even years after the illness. Pathological evidence also indicates the unity of the two conditions.

Proof that the Wernicke-Korsakoff syndrome is due to thiamin deficiency and not to chronic alcohol intoxication is shown by the fact that the condition responds to thiamin alone, even if the patient continues to consume alcohol.

Of overriding importance in this syndrome is the fact that irreversible brain damage ensues rapidly; early recognition and treatment are therefore vital. If there is any suspicion that a patient may have the syndrome, he should immediately receive 5 to 10 mg of thiamin by injection, even before a definitive diagnosis is made.

Prevention: The prevention of the Wernicke-Korsakoff syndrome calls for considerable public health ingenuity. Several possible measures have been suggested[37]:

a The "immunization" of alcoholics with large doses of thiamin at regular intervals. (The development of a suitable depot carrier to reduce the frequency of these injections would be very helpful.)

b The fortification of alcoholic beverages with thiamin.

c A provision by public health authorities that thiamin-impregnated snacks be available on bar counters.

The cost of any of these measures would almost certainly be less than is the present enormous expenditure on institutional care of those who have suffered from Wernicke-Korsakoff disease.

Other Thiamin-Deficiency States

Alcoholic polyneuropathy, a condition similar to neuritic beriberi, is also due to a dietary deficiency of thiamin.

An optic or retrobulbar neuritis that occurred in prison camps during World War II was probably due to thiamin deficiency. The condition, also known as nutritional amblyopia, was at least in part due to thiamin deficiency.

PELLAGRA

Pellagra, which was once common in the southern United States, is now seldom seen in this country. The disease is associated with a corn (maize) diet and is primarily due to a dietary deficiency of niacin, one of the B-complex vitamins. Although there is more niacin in corn than in some other staple foods, the vitamin is evidently not completely utilized, most likely because it is in a bound form unavailable to

Figure 20A. Casal's necklace– advanced pellagra. Dermatitis outlining the exposed area of the neck is pathognomonic of pellagra, as are the character- istic lesions on the backs of the hands. Either sunlight or heat from a stove may have been the precipitating factor.

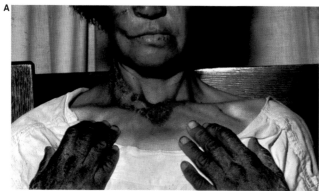

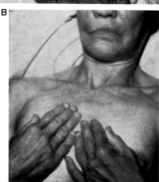

Figure 20B. Same patient after nicotinamide therapy.

the body. The human body can convert the amino acid trypto- phan into niacin, so a high-protein diet rich in tryptophan will help prevent pellagra. The main protein in corn is zein, which is very low in tryptophan content.

The Disease

To the medical student, pellagra is portrayed by "the four Ds" – dermatitis, diarrhea, dementia, and death. The disease is most often diagnosed from the characteristic appearance of the skin lesions. These lesions are often symmetrical in appearance and occur on areas of the body exposed to sun- light such as the face, the neck, and the forearms. In whites, the skin lesions at first resemble the erythema of sunburn. In blacks, there is a hyperpigmentation. The affected areas become dry, scaly, and cracked, and if the condition progresses, desquamation commonly occurs. There may be cracking and fissuring, and occasionally the skin becomes blistered. In persons who usually wear open-neck shirts, the upper chest and lower neck are affected; the lesion is known as Casal's necklace (Figure 20).

Digestive symptoms include abdominal pain and diarrhea. Frequently, the tongue and mouth are sore, and angular sto- matitis and cheilosis, usually associated with riboflavin deficiency, sometimes occur (Figure 21). The tongue is often red, smooth, and raw looking (Figure 22).

Involvement of the nervous system manifests itself by ex- tremely variable symptoms and signs. The commonest of these are irritability, loss of memory, insomnia, and anxiety. These may lead to dementia. It was once common for persons to be incarcerated in mental institutions without anyone realizing that their mental condition was due to pellagra. In areas where corn is the primary staple food, all persons admitted to mental institutions should be examined for evi- dence of pellagra.

Mild sensory and motor changes occasionally occur in pellagra, but paralysis is very rare.

Diagnosis

Pellagra is usually diagnosed on the basis of the dietary his- tory and on physical examination.

Treatment

Hospital admission is necessary only for very serious cases. The basis of treatment is niacinamide, 50 to 100 mg three times daily by intramuscular injection for the first three to four days and subsequently by mouth. A high-caloric diet including at least 100 gm of high-quality protein is recommended.

If the patient has abdominal burning or diarrhea, an easily digestible diet low in fiber content should be given. Sedation is recommended for the first few days of treatment. Those with mental disturbances benefit greatly from a tranquilizer prescribed in relatively large doses. A vitamin B complex preparation is useful to counteract concurrent deficiencies of other B vitamins.

SCURVY

Scurvy is a rare disease today. It results from a deficiency of vitamin C and usually occurs only after considerable time in persons on a diet containing very little fresh fruit or vegetables. Daily intakes of vitamin C considerably less than the recommended allowances, even for periods of several months, usually do not result in scurvy.

Vitamin C is necessary for the formation and healthy upkeep of intercellular material. In scurvy, the walls of the capillaries lack solidity and become fragile, resulting in hemorrhage from various sites.

The Disease

Scurvy is characterized by the following symptoms and signs:
a Tenderness of the extremities, muscle weakness, and suppressed appetite may be evident.
b Gums become swollen and bleed easily; teeth may become loose.
c Hemorrhages of a petechial type often occur in the skin.
d Hemorrhages in other areas may manifest themselves as nose bleeds, hematuria, melena, splinter hemorrhages below the nails, and painful subperiosteal hemorrhages.
e Delayed healing of wounds and heightened risk of infection may occur.
f Anemia and shortness of breath may be noted.

A patient with scurvy and some of the above symptoms and signs, though not appearing very seriously ill, may suddenly collapse and die of cardiac failure.

Infantile Scurvy (Barlow's Disease)

Infantile scurvy typically occurs in infants 2 to 12 months of age who are bottle fed with a milk formula unsupplemented by vitamin C and who do not receive any other source of vitamin C. The vitamin C in milk is destroyed by heat in the process of pasteurization or drying.

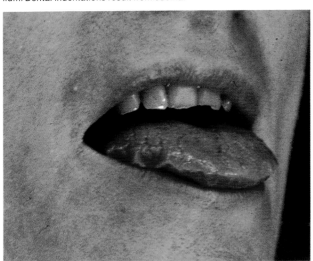

Figure 21. Glossitis is the earliest diagnostic sign of pellagra brought about by nicotinamide deficiency. It starts with a burning sensation, which is followed either by edema or by desquamation of the epithelium. Dental indentations result from edema.

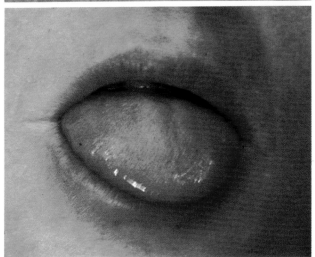

Figure 22. The tip and margins of the tongue are made scarlet red and shiny by desquamation of the epithelium. There are signs of healed angular stomatitis, indicating a previous riboflavin deficiency.

Figure 23. Infant with scurvy in the "pithed frog" position. Because movement is painful, the scorbutic infant usually lies on its back and makes little attempt to lift the leg or arm that hurts. Both legs may be tender, and sometimes both arms as well. This is usually the first sign of scurvy.

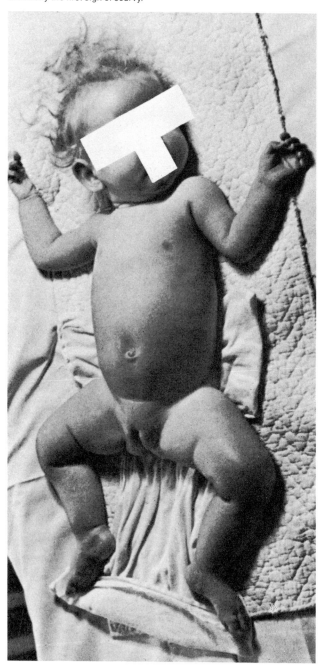

The infant with scurvy cries when the limbs are touched or moved, because of pain and tenderness. The infant often lies with his limbs placed in what has been called the "pithed frog" position (Figure 23). Swelling due to hemorrhages may be felt especially in the legs, and there may be obvious bruising of the body. Hemorrhages may occur from any of the sites mentioned previously for adult scurvy, except that gum bleeding does not occur unless there are erupted teeth.

Diagnosis of Scurvy

The capillary fragility test is useful, but conditions other than scurvy also influence capillary strength. Estimations of ascorbic acid content in serum, or preferably in white blood cells, may be useful. If ascorbic acid is present, the disease is not scurvy. Decreased urinary excretion of ascorbic acid is an early sign. Roentgenograms aid in the diagnosis of infantile scurvy; in older patients, the presence of "scurvy lines" of the tibia and femur are useful in diagnosis.

The concentration of ascorbic acid in the blood plasma reflects the dietary intake and does not indicate the degree of depletion of the bodily stores. It is better to measure the concentration of ascorbic acid in the leukocytes. Concentrations less than 2 mg/dl provide presumptive evidence of scurvy.

Treatment

Because of the danger of sudden death, even in the patient who looks reasonably well, there is a need for immediate vigorous treatment. It is advisable to give a loading dose of 1 gm ascorbic acid, orally, followed by 250 mg four times daily for six to seven days; the dosage can then usually be reduced to 50 mg twice a day until recovery is complete. The patient should also be given a diet containing plenty of fresh fruit and vegetables. The ascorbic acid must be given by injection if the patient is vomiting, and the injectable form is also useful in treating infants.

RICKETS AND OSTEOMALACIA

In both rickets and osteomalacia, there is a lack of calcium retention in the skeleton. The conditions are, however, due mainly to a deficiency of vitamin D and not of dietary calcium. Vitamin D is obtained both from the diet and from exposure of the skin to sunlight. The average unsupplemented diet contains only relatively small amounts of vitamin D, but nowadays the vitamin is added to many processed foods, especially those commonly consumed by young children. Vitamin D deficiency is therefore uncommon in children and is very rare in adults in the United States.

Rickets – The Disease

Unlike the child with any of a number of other deficiency diseases, the child with rickets often has the superficial appearance of being plump and well fed. The child's appearance frequently gives the mother a false sense of security. The story has often been told of the rachitic child winning the baby show because it appeared so fat and well nourished (Figure 24). The child, however, tends to be miserable, and closer examination will reveal the flabby toneless state of the muscles. Another feature is the general impairment of normal development. The child is frequently late in reaching all the milestones in his early life; he is slow to learn, to sit, to walk, and to get his teeth. Other generalized signs include gastrointestinal upsets and excessive sweating of the head.

The main signs of the disease – those by which the diagnosis of rickets is made – are the skeletal changes. One early feature is swelling of the epiphysis of the long bones. This may first be found at the wrist, where the radius is enlarged. Another classical site is at the costochondral junctions, where swelling produces the bead-like appearance that has been called "rachitic rosary." Deformities of the chest lead to the formation of Harrison's sulcus and pigeon breast. Swellings of the epiphyses of the tibia, fibula, and femur may also be seen.

In young infants, the first sign of rickets is often craniotabes, which consists of areas of softening of the skull, usually affecting the occipital and parietal bones. There is also delayed closing of the anterior fontanel. In severe rickets there may be bossing of the skull.

When a child with rickets begins to stand and walk, he often develops new deformities because of the soft, weak character of the bones. The commonest deformity is bowlegs (Figures 25 and 26); knock-knees are seen less frequently. More serious, however, are spinal deformities that lead to kyphosis. Changes in the pelvis, though often not obvious, may cause the woman who had rickets during her childhood to have difficulty during childbirth.

Tetany due to a reduction in the level of serum calcium sometimes occurs. It presents an unmistakable picture with spasm of the hands, the thumb being drawn into the palm.

Diagnosis: Radiologic examination will reveal abnormali-

Figure 24. Two girls with rickets: The cases of Ethel and Evelyn.

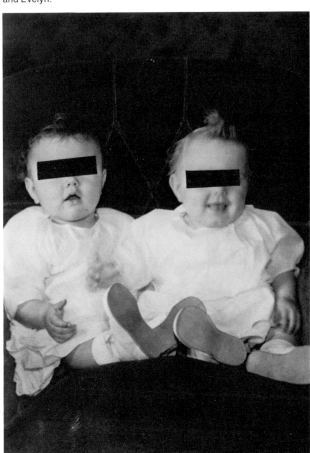

These patients, twins, were first seen on July 10, two days after they had won first prize at a baby show. Both infants were female and appeared to be well nourished. They were markedly obese. On physical examination, there was a definite craniotabes. The anterior fontanel was open. There was a flaring of the lower rib margin and a well-marked rachitic rosary. There was an extreme bowing of both legs, which was more marked in the lower third (see Figure 26A).

These children had been raised on artificial feeding with no supplemental vitamin D. They were placed on high doses of vitamin D concentrate. A very rapid improvement was noted in both cases, especially that of Ethel, whose condition was so severe that she was placed in bed with traction on both feet. We were not able to secure x-ray films again until February 7 (see Figure 26B). At that time there was an increase in the density of the bone with a marked thickening of the cortex of the shaft on the concave side. The epiphyseal line is much narrower and the margin is much more regular in outline.

44

Figure 25. Child with bowlegs due to rickets. The child's family is moderately well-to-do.

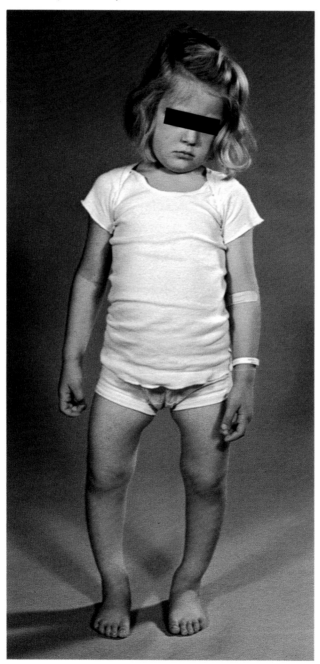

Figure 26A. 7-10-35, Roentgenologic findings (right and left legs and ankles): X-ray films of the legs and ankles show a marked flaring and widening of the diaphysis above the epiphyseal line. The zone between the shaft and epiphysis is increased in thickness with ragged fringy margins. There is a marked bowing of the lower end of the tibia.
Conclusion– Rachitic infant

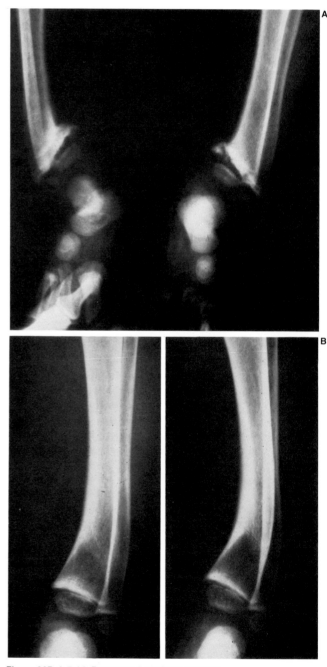

Figure 26B. 2-7-36, Roentgenologic findings (right and left legs and ankles). X-ray films after treatment show an increase in the density of the bone. There is a marked thickening of the cortex of the shaft on the concave side. The epiphyseal line is much narrower and the margin is much more regular in outline. Conclusion– X-ray films show a marked improvement.

ties and is also helpful in showing progress during treatment. Roentgenograms, especially of the wrists, but also of the ends of long bones at other sites, are useful in diagnosis. The films will usually reveal characteristic changes in the epiphyses (Figure 27). The outline of the joint is blurred, the epiphyseal line is broadened, and later the end of the bone shaft appears saucered. The trabeculation of the bone becomes coarse and there is a decrease in bone density. Curvature of bones may be even more evident by roentgenography than by clinical examination, especially in a plump child. Some of the early radiologic signs of rickets are rather similar to those of infantile scurvy.

The serum alkaline phosphatase concentration is usually elevated well above the normal range of 5 to 15 Bodansky units. A level above 20 units in a child is very suggestive of rickets. The serum phosphorus concentration is usually reduced to 2 to 4 mg/dl (normal = 4.5 to 5.5 mg/dl), but the serum calcium is frequently normal or only slightly reduced, being around 10 mg/dl.

Treatment: The basis of treatment is the provision of adequate quantities of vitamin D and at the same time ensuring an adequate intake of calcium. A vitamin preparation that provides about 75 μg (300 IU) of vitamin D daily is the recommended therapy. Calcium supplementation is usually given as milk.

While the child is being treated, the mother should be educated about the value of sunshine on the body and about good nutrition.

Mild bony deformities tend to right themselves following dietary treatment, but in more-serious cases some degree of deformity may persist.

Osteomalacia – The Disease

Osteomalacia is the adult counterpart of rickets and has the same general causes. It occurs much more frequently in women than in men. It is most common in women on a poor diet who have been depleted of calcium by many years of pregnancies and lactation, who get very little vitamin D in their diet, and who are protected from the sun by their clothing and confinement indoors. The condition is usually very rare in the United States.

Pain occurs in the bones of the pelvis, lower back, and legs. Tenderness may be elicited by pressure on the affected bones. Deformities occur later, especially in the pelvis and spine. The patient may walk with his feet widely spaced and may

Figure 27A. Rickets in a 3-month-old infant.

Figure 27B. Healing after 28 days of vitamin D treatment.

Figure 27C. After 41 days. In these photographs no shadow is cast by the epiphyses, which are still unossified.

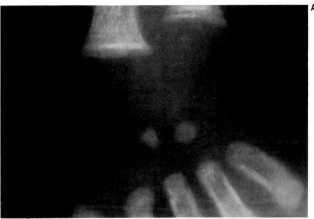

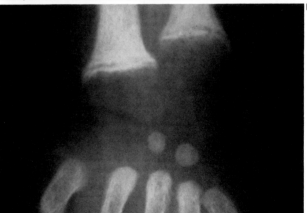

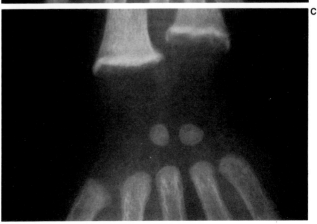

Figure 28. Goiter in a young woman.

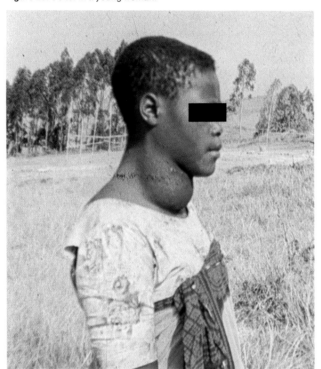

appear to waddle. Spontaneous fractures often are a complication of severe osteomalacia. In some cases, tetany develops and may be seen as involuntary twitchings of the muscles of the face and as carpopedal spasms.

Diagnosis: Roentgenograms will show extensive demineralization, bony deformities, and, if present, fractures. The concentration of serum alkaline phosphatase is raised above the maximum normal adult level of 5 Bodansky units, and the concentration of serum calcium is often decreased below 8 mg/dl.

Treatment: Vitamin D, 125 μg (50,000 IU) daily, should be given as a vitamin preparation. Calcium is easily provided as milk, if available; otherwise some other form such as calcium lactate is adequate. Exposure of the skin to sunlight should be encouraged. Good obstetrical care is very important in women who have pelvic abnormalities due to osteomalacia.

ENDEMIC GOITER

Goiter is the name used for any swelling of the thyroid gland. When it occurs sporadically it may be due to any of various causes not related to diet and, therefore, not relevant to this monograph.[38] However, where goiter is common or endemic in a district or in a community, the cause is usually nutritional, due to a lack of the mineral nutrient iodide.

In endemic goiter areas, many people have some enlargement of the thyroid gland and a smaller number have large and obvious swellings of the neck (Figures 28 and 29). By far the commonest cause of endemic goiter is a deficiency of iodide in the diet of those affected. The amount of iodide present in soil varies from place to place, and the soil content affects the quantity both in food grown and in the water supply of the area. Seafoods such as fish, shellfish, and seaweed are rich sources of iodide. Endemic goiter areas are usually far from the sea.

Experiments with animals have shown that certain foods eaten in large quantities make the animal more liable to develop goiter even if normal quantities of iodide are consumed. Substances with that effect are called goitrogens and are known to exist in certain varieties of cabbage, kale, turnips, and some other vegetables. There is little evidence to incriminate dietary goitrogens as being important in endemic goiter in man.

In the United States, endemic areas of goiter are mainly in the states bordering on Canada (especially in the Great Lakes area) and those states between the Rocky Mountains and the Appalachians.

Figure 29. Advanced nodular goiters in an endemic area in Tanzania.

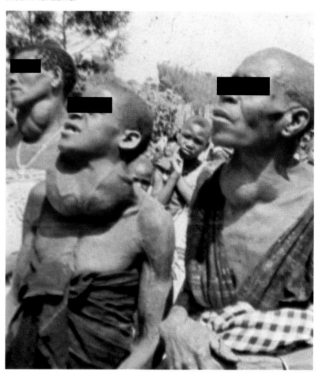

Physiology of Endemic Goiter

The thyroid gland requires iodide to produce thyroxine, which contains 64% iodide. When iodide is deficient, the gland enlarges to compensate for the difficulty in producing thyroxine. This basically is the mechanism at work in goiter due to iodide deficiency.

The normal thyroid gland contains about 8 mg of iodide, and this may be reduced to 1 to 2 mg in persons with goiter. The thyroid gland is under the control of the anterior pituitary gland. Iodide is absorbed from the intestines at a rate dependent on thyroid activity. The rate of secretion of thyroid-stimulating hormone (TSH) by the anterior pituitary depends upon the concentration of thyroid hormones circulating in the blood. Thyroxine administration will therefore inhibit TSH secretion.

The iodide uptake in normal persons is proportional to the blood concentration of the thyroid hormones. It has been shown that the uptake of radioactive iodide is increased in hyperthyroidism and decreased in hypothyroidism. There are, however, other factors that can influence it.

The total iodide content of whole blood is usually 10 μg $\pm$ 4 μg, of which 6 μg $\pm$ 2μg is protein bound. The protein bound iodide (PBI) is reduced in hypothyroidism and elevated in hyperthyroidism. The amount of iodide in the urine depends mainly on the dietary intake of iodide and on thyroid activity.

Endemic goiter is diagnosed when there is thyroid enlargement in a patient who lives in an area where endemic goiter is known to occur, where there is evidence that the iodide intake of the patient is low, and where other causes of thyroid enlargement can be ruled out.

Urinary excretion of iodide in patients with endemic goiter is usually less than 100 μg daily, the protein bound iodide is in the normal range, and the uptake of the radioactive isotope ^{131}I is often increased.

Goiter Surveys

When the prevalence of goiter in a population is being studied, the thyroid glands of a representative sample should be examined both visually and by palpation in order to estimate the degree of enlargement. Each lobe of the normal thyroid gland is about the size of the thumbnail of the person being examined. The World Health Organization has suggested the following classifications of goiter size (Figure 30)[39]:

Group 0 – Persons without goiter and persons whose thyroids are less than five times enlarged

Figure 30. Classification of goiters. Neck profiles illustrating categories of thyroid enlargement.

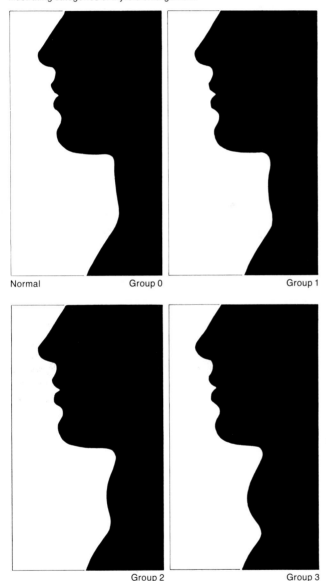

Normal   Group 0   Group 1

Group 2   Group 3

Group 1 – Persons whose thyroids are more than five times enlarged but which are not easily visible when the patient's head is in a normal (ie, upright, forward-looking) position
Group 2 – Persons who have goiters that are easily visible even when the head is in a normal position but smaller than those seen in Group 3
Group 3 – Persons who have large goiters that can be easily recognized at a considerable distance and that may be disfiguring

The Disease

Goiter is more common among females, particularly at puberty and during pregnancy. The enlargement of the gland may be smooth and is then said to be a colloid goiter, or it may be lumpy and is then called an adenomatous or nodular goiter.

Endemic goiter, in which there is a benign enlargement of the thyroid gland, may cause no symptoms. The enlargement is merely evidence of a deficient intake of iodide. Appropriate treatment will prevent both further enlargement and the complications that may accompany goiter and, in many cases, will cause the gland to return to its normal size. Untreated, the gland may enlarge to a size that is obvious and presents a cosmetic problem. Further enlargement may produce pressure symptoms such as difficulty in breathing, persistent cough, or voice changes. A person with a simple goiter may develop the symptoms and signs of hyperthyroidism. Carcinoma of the thyroid is more common among those with goiters.

Cretinism in children occurs most commonly in endemic goiter areas and is usually due to severe iodide deficiency of the mother. The infant might appear normal at birth but is slow to develop, small in size, mentally dull, and has thick skin and characteristic facial features such as a depressed nose and, often, a protruding, enlarged tongue. Deaf mutism and mental retardation are common among the children of mothers with enlarged thyroid glands.

Treatment

Small diffuse colloid goiters will reduce in size and may disappear with suitable iodide therapy or with an increased dietary intake of iodide. The recommended treatment is Lugol's solution of iodide, 0.5 ml in water per day by mouth.

More-dramatic improvement, especially in those with larger goiters, can be achieved by the use of thyroid extract or thyroxine. If this form of therapy is used, the weight, pulse rate, and, if possible, the basal metabolic rate of the patient should be checked at regular intervals. Treatment should start with a small dose, eg, thyroid extract ½ gr daily, and increased gradually to 2 gr daily. Weight loss, increased pulse rate, and an elevated BMR are indications of hyperthyroidism and are a signal to reduce the dosage.

Surgical treatment consisting of subtotal thyroidectomy is indicated for large goiters, especially the adenomatous type and for those exceptional cases that do not respond to iodide or thyroid extract.

Prevention of Endemic Goiter

Where goiter is prevalent it constitutes a public health problem and should be tackled as such. The most satisfactory measure is the addition of iodide to all salt sold in the area. Use of the salt will reduce the size of many existing goiters and will prevent most goiters from developing in the future.

Salt is iodized most commonly with sodium or potassium iodide to a level that provides about 0.5 gm of iodide to 1 kg of salt. The less-volatile potassium iodate is preferable to iodide for iodization in hot, humid countries or regions. When endemic goiter is a problem, legislation is desirable to ensure that all salt is iodized. Unfortunately, legislation does not now exist throughout the United States, or even in most states, to require the iodization of all table salt or salt used in processed foods. Iodized and noniodized salt are displayed side-by-side in stores.

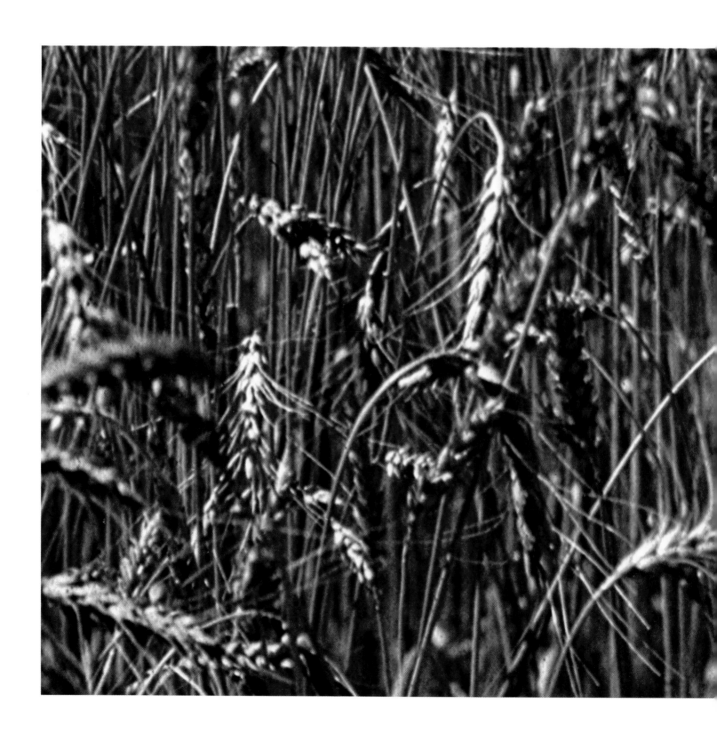

Nutrients

PROTEIN

Dietary proteins furnish the necessary sources of amino acids and nitrogen for synthesis of body proteins and the array of other nitrogen-containing compounds (except the nitrogen-containing vitamins). Most of the dietary protein is used as amino acids and absorbed by the intestinal mucosa after hydrolysis of complex peptide chains. About 22 amino acids are biologically important. Of these, eight so-called essential amino acids cannot be synthesized by human beings in amounts necessary for their needs.[40] These are lysine, leucine, isoleucine, methionine, phenylalanine, threonine, tryptophan, and valine. In addition, an exogenous supply of histidine is necessary for early growth and development. It is not clear whether histidine is required in the adult, but since no biosynthetic path for this amino acid has been found in humans, it probably is. Requirements for the other amino acids are met either through exogenous sources or through endogenous sources by means of synthesis from appropriate metabolic precursors and exogenous amino nitrogen.

The fetal liver cannot convert methionine to cysteine, and premature infants are known to require cysteine. Although premature infants are able to convert phenylalanine into tyrosine, the latter becomes an essential amino acid in phenylketonuria, an inborn error of metabolism in which the enzyme phenylalanine hydroxylase is absent. An interesting amino acid that is not found in proteins but which plays an important role in the central nervous system, retina, and heart is taurine.[41] Most species can synthesize taurine from methionine, but human beings have a very limited ability to do so, and it is conjectured that premature infants may require exogenous taurine.

Dietary proteins are supplied by both animal and plant materials. The nutritional quality of proteins from various sources is a function of the particular amino acids they contain in relation to essential amino acid requirements.

In general, protein from animal sources is of greater nutritional value because it contains all of the essential amino acids plus the nonessential ones. Proteins from cereals and vegetables are relatively deficient in certain amino acids, particularly lysine, tryptophan, threonine, and methionine, depending on the specific cereal or vegetable. In addition, cereal and vegetable proteins provide fewer of all the essential amino acids per unit weight than do proteins from animal sources. On the other hand, relatively small amounts of a high-quality animal protein can efficiently supplement the relative amino acid deficiencies in diets obtained mainly from plant protein. Similarly, appropriate mixtures of cereals, legumes, or other vegetable foods may have a protein quality approaching that of animal foods.

Undoubtedly, protein quality is of great importance in rapidly growing young animals, which are actively depositing new body protein. On the other hand, adult animals have lesser requirements both for total protein (per kg of body weight) and for essential amino acids (per gm of protein). Thus, the World Health Organization believes that a newborn infant needs dietary protein that contains 37% of its weight in the form of essential amino acids, whereas for adults the figure is less than half – about 15%. This has led many to suspect that protein quality is of limited relevance to adults. Indeed, it can be argued that after the first year of life, protein quality is of little importance.[42]

Digestion of amino acids proceeds to the stage of a mixture of amino acids and dipeptides and tripeptides. It is now clear that a considerable part of dietary protein is absorbed in the form of short peptides that are hydrolyzed in the mucosal cells.[43] This absorption occurs by means of a system independent of that by which amino acids are absorbed. The amino acids themselves are absorbed by an active transport system against a concentration gradient. Specificities in the transfer sites lead to differential rates of absorption and to competition in the transport of amino acids across the intestinal mucosa. A similar transfer system operates in other cells as well. There is no known "pool" – in the usual metabolic sense – of amino acids. And so a continuing, normal level of protein synthesis requires the continuous availability of the entire array of necessary amino acids. The removal of even one essential amino acid from the diet leads rather rapidly to a lower level of protein synthesis in the body.

Minimal protein requirements for a healthy adult represent the sum of the requirements for the essential amino acids plus sufficient utilizable nitrogen to maintain overall synthesis of nitrogen-containing molecules. Nitrogen is lost in urine, feces, skin, hair, and nails. Though there are considerable problems in measuring minimal protein requirement, it is of the order of 0.3 to 0.4 gm of protein/kg/day, assuming a reasonable amount of high-quality protein of an appropriate mixture of cereal or vegetable protein with an adequate level of overall calories. With lower-quality proteins, greater quantities are required to maintain nitrogen balance. Early growth and development, pregnancy, lactation, and periods of physical stress add to the basal requirements for protein. Recommended allowances include a twofold-to-threefold "safety factor" over minimal requirements and apply to the ranges of quality in mixed proteins ordinarily consumed.

It is the very high (on a body-weight basis) requirement for protein during early growth and development that makes this age group especially vulnerable to dietary deprivation.

In addition, the sometimes very marked degradation of protein and excretion of urinary nitrogen that accompany the stress of even ordinarily mild childhood illnesses put such an added burden on an already tenuously nourished infant that the condition can deteriorate to frank, clinical malnutrition.

The main sources of protein in the industrialized countries are animal products (meat, fish, and poultry; milk and its products; and eggs), which in the United States account for about 75% of the protein intake. Other significant sources of protein in the Eastern countries are cereal grains and legumes.

Because of the prohibitive cost of animal protein in the developing countries, cereals (and, to a lesser extent, legumes) are by far the greatest source of protein.

CARBOHYDRATES

Carbohydrates comprise the major energy source for populations throughout the world and, being derived from foods readily and efficiently grown in nearly all climates, are cheaper than animal proteins and fats. The carbohydrate contribution to total daily calories is about 45% in the diets of people in highly developed areas, whereas for the 85% of the world's population that rely mainly on plants as sources of food, this contribution amounts to about 70% and may be as high as 90%.

The common hexoses – glucose, fructose, galactose, and mannose – are the digestive products absorbed from the gastrointestinal hydrolysis of the disaccharides and polysaccharides present in foods.

In affluent societies, half to two thirds of dietary carbohydrate is furnished by starches, about a quarter by sucrose, and the rest is provided by lactose, glucose, fructose, and partly digestible polysaccharides. Refined sugar, by which is generally meant sucrose, provides in adult diets about 25% of the total carbohydrate – 10% to 15% of the total daily calories. In the diets of children, sucrose is generally more prevalent, approaching half of the total carbohydrate, or 20% to 25% of the total calories. Even then, at least 75% of total calories are from sources other than sugar. In lesser-developed areas the types of carbohydrate are different. Sucrose and lactose are consumed in smaller quantities, while starches make up most of the carbohydrate. A trend in American diets is the decreasing consumption of starches. Per capita consumption of sucrose has been quite constant. Cereals, fruits, and vegetables contribute to the vitamin and mineral intake in diets in which they provide the major source of calories. In American diets the increased use of refined carbohydrates may produce constraints on the achievement of adequate nutrient intakes in diets very low in calories. For example, in diets of 1,000 Calories or less, the proportions of sucrose, other refined sugars, and fats should be reduced to ensure adequate intake of other nutrients from foods consumed. However, about 75% of the sugar and most of the fat one consumes are as constituents of foods that do contain other nutrients, so one obtains nutrients other than sugar and fat from those foods.

No specific requirements for type, source, or amount of carbohydrates have been established. During starvation and with calorie-restricted diets, carbohydrates serve to spare body proteins for energy purposes; as little as 100 gm per day (400 Calories) of carbohydrates can prevent the water and electrolyte loss that attends protein catabolism, and probably as little as 40 gm per day will prevent the development of ketosis.

FATS

Fats and oils in nutrition have historically been associated with the energy or caloric value of a diet and with its satiety value. This is because they provide, per unit of weight, twice the number of calories of either carbohydrate or protein (9 Calories per gm versus 4) and because most people enjoy the taste of fats as they are characteristically used in our diets. Because fats remain in the stomach appreciably longer than do carbohydrates or proteins, they tend to give a feeling of "gastronomic satisfaction" for a somewhat longer period of time. More recently, the interest in fats has been concerned less with their caloric and satiety properties and more with their influence on the level of cholesterol in the blood and their association with atherosclerosis.

About 98% of dietary fats are triglycerides, compounds of glycerol and specific fatty acids. Since glycerol has three hydroxyl groups, each of which can combine with a fatty acid, we speak of triglycerides, diglycerides, and monoglycerides, depending upon how many of the hydroxyl groups of the glycerol molecule have been esterified with a fatty acid. Additionally, these fatty acids may be saturated, monounsaturated, or polyunsaturated. The term "saturation" refers to the degree of hydrogenation of the carbon atoms of the fatty-acid chain. When the maximum number of hydrogen atoms is attached to the carbon atoms of the fatty-acid chain, the chain is "saturated" with hydrogen – a saturated fat. If the carbon chain has one double bond and hence can accept two more hydrogen atoms, we call the fat "monounsaturated." If the carbon chain has two or more double bonds and thus can accept four or more hydrogen atoms, we call the fat "polyunsaturated." As previously stated, all naturally occurring fats are mixtures of saturated, monounsaturated, and polyunsaturated fats, but the mixtures vary widely in composition. Thus, butter averages 66% saturates, 31% monounsaturates, and 3% polyunsaturates. Soybean oil averages 15% saturates, 25% monounsaturates, and 60% polyunsaturates; safflower and sunflower oils have a still higher percentage of polyunsaturates (approximately 75%) and correspondingly lower proportions of monounsaturates and saturates.

In the processes of digestion, fats are hydrolyzed into diglycerides, monoglycerides, and fatty acids mostly by the action of various enzymes – lipases. Because these lipases are present in pancreatic and intestinal juices, most of the digestion of fat takes place in the upper part of the small intestine. In the small intestine, the fats are emulsified by the bile, and this process facilitates the enzymatic action of the various lipases. Ordinarily, most 12-carbon and longer fatty acids, upon being emulsified and hydrolyzed, are absorbed into the lymphatic system and transported in association with cholesterol, phospholipids, and protein; these particles are termed chylomicrons. The chylomicrons then undergo a process of dissolution brought about by the action of an enzyme, lipoprotein lipase, found in blood and tissue. Shorter-chain fatty acids, in contrast, are absorbed directly into the portal blood, where they are found as free fatty acids. These short-chain free fatty acids are a very minor component of all foods other than dairy products.

In recent years, finely divided and stable emulsions of fat have been prepared, which may be given intravenously. Such emulsions are metabolized similarly to consumed fat, and they serve a useful role when complete intravenous nutrition is necessary for periods of several weeks.

Because the level of cholesterol in the blood is one of the factors associated with the development of coronary heart disease and other manifestations of atherosclerosis, and because the type of dietary fat is an important factor influencing the level of cholesterol in the blood, interest in fat has greatly increased in recent years. In general, the saturated fats increase the level of blood cholesterol, the monounsaturated fats have no effect, and the polyunsaturated fats decrease the cholesterol level. There is as yet no clear biochemical explanation for these regulating effects. The common saturated fats of our diet are meat fat, milk fat, butter, cream, most cheeses, and coconut and palm oils. Olive and peanut oils are examples of oils in which the predominant fats are monounsaturated. Soya, corn, cottonseed, sunflower, and safflower oils are the common oils in which the predominant fat is polyunsaturated because of the linoleic acid they contain. A diet designed to lower the level of cholesterol in the blood is low in total calories and saturated fat and is high in unsaturated fat, particularly polyunsaturated fat (see section on cardiovascular disease, page 16).

The four commonly used polyunsaturated vegetable oils average 50% or more linoleic acid (safflower and sunflower oils are about 75% linoleic acid). In the preparation of these oils for commercial use in products such as shortenings and margarine, and to give the oils greater stability, they are partially hydrogenated. This, of course, reduces their polyunsaturation and increases their saturation. But hydrogenation is a controllable process. One can hydrogenate a lot or a little. Thus, a vegetable oil, 50% of which consisted of the polyunsaturated fatty acid, linoleic, may have been hydrogenated in the process of making margarine so that the polyunsaturation has been reduced to 35%, for example; the final product is nevertheless still a good source of linoleic acid, as compared with lard at about 9% polyunsaturates and with butter at less than 3% of polyunsaturates.

Another dietary fat component that influences the level of blood lipids is dietary cholesterol. The level of consumption of egg yolk, butterfat, and meat fats in the usual American diet provides from 600 to 800 mg daily of exogenous cholesterol, with egg yolks alone contributing two thirds of the total. Foods rich in cholesterol (such as egg yolks) are also restricted in planning fat-modified diets. Egg whites are devoid of cholesterol and are essentially pure protein of the highest nutritional quality.

There is no dietary requirement for either saturated or monounsaturated fatty acids, both of which are easily synthesized by the body. Polyunsaturated fatty acids cannot be synthesized and must therefore be provided by the diet. The daily requirement is, however, small (about 1% to 2% of calories); deficiencies do not develop in those who eat normally, but they may develop in patients undergoing prolonged intravenous feeding.

In addition to their role in cholesterol metabolism, polyunsaturated fatty acids play a role in membrane stability and are precursors of prostaglandins, a group of compounds that exhibit many important physiological functions.

WATER

Because water forms nearly 70% of the body weight of man, it obviously plays an important part in metabolism. Except for fat storage, the whole series of chemical actions that are intimately related to the life of a living organism, animal or vegetable, are ultimately referable to changes that take place in solution. It has been shown that the younger the animal, the richer it is in water. It has also been found that the fatter the animal, the smaller the percentage of water.

Water serves as a solvent to help absorb water-soluble nutrients and eliminate water-soluble waste products via the urine. Water is indispensable for the control of body temperature by means of evaporation from the lungs and from the skin.

Water furnishes no calories or vitamins, but it may provide various minerals – calcium and magnesium in hard water, and fluoride in waters that have been fluoridated either naturally or by man.

The minimum daily water requirement in a temperate climate is about 2 liters, of which about 50 to 90 dl is required for the excretion (at maximal concentration) of waste products, about 10 dl is lost in stools, and slightly more than a liter is lost through the skin and lungs (even in the absence of visible sweating). Requirements can increase enormously with profuse sweating, and pathological losses due to vomiting or diarrhea must, of course, be replaced.

Water is available to the body not only simply as water that one drinks, plain or in beverages, but also in foods, even those that seem dry. Not surprisingly, many fruits have a water content of 80% to 90%; yet even bread, which appears to be dry, is about 35% water. Finally, small amounts of water are formed in the body from the oxidation of food.

MINERALS
Iron
The average iron content of a healthy adult is only about 4 gm, and yet this relatively small quantity is vitally important.[44] Iron-deficiency anemia is a common cause of ill health in the United States and in all parts of the world.

About two thirds of the iron in the body is present in the blood mainly as hemoglobin, and approximately 35% is present as myoglobin. Most of the remainder is storage iron in the form of ferritin or hemosiderin in the liver, spleen, bone marrow, and muscle. Additional minute quantities exist in the respiratory enzymes and in iron-binding protein of the plasma.

The main function of iron is its vital role in the transfer of oxygen at various sites in the body. Iron is an essential component of hemoglobin, the pigment in the erythrocytes that carries oxygen from the lungs to the tissues. Iron is present as myoglobin in skeletal and heart muscle (where it functions by accepting the oxygen from the hemoglobin) and also in peroxidase, catalase, and the cytochromes.

Iron is an element that is neither used up nor destroyed in the properly functioning body. Unlike some minerals it is not required for excretion, and only very small amounts appear in the urine and sweat. Minute quantities are lost in desquamated cells from the skin and intestine, in shed hair and nails, and in the bile and other body secretions. The body is, however, efficiently economical and conservative in the use of iron. Iron released when the erythrocytes are old and broken down is taken up and used again and again for the manufacture of new erythrocytes. This economy with iron is important. In normal circumstances, only about 1 mg of iron is lost to the body daily by excretion into the intestines, in urine, in sweat, or through loss of hair or surface epithelial cells.

Because iron is preserved, the nutritional needs of healthy males and postmenopausal females are very small. Women of childbearing age must, however, make good the iron lost during menstruation and childbirth and must meet the additional requirements of pregnancy and lactation. Children have relatively high needs because of their rapid growth, which increases not only their body size but also their blood volume.

Sources of iron: Iron is present in a variety of foods of both plant and animal origin. In many foods there is considerable variation in the value of iron content, depending on the soil and conditions in which the food is raised. Rich food sources for iron include meat (especially liver), egg yolk, and pulses such as beans and peas. However, many other common foods such as green leafy vegetables, whole-grain and enriched cereals, vegetables, and fish are also good sources of iron. Milk, both human and cow's, contrary to the notion that it is the "perfect food," is a poor source of iron.

In the United States, many prepared foods such as bread, breakfast cereals, and certain baby foods are artificially enriched with iron. An average American adult diet consisting of a variety of common foods bought at a grocery store or eaten in a restaurant or institution would normally contain about 15 mg of iron per day. Because of the poor absorption of iron, that may be a rather marginal amount for women in the child-bearing years.

Many studies in which the iron content of a diet was calculated from food composition tables and then actually measured by chemical analysis have shown far more iron to be present than had been expected. The usual explanation is that the extra iron has come from cooking utensils, and the amount of iron so added to the food seems to depend upon the acidity of the food and the duration of cooking. The shift from cast-iron cookware to stainless steel or aluminum has led to a decrease in the available iron in our diets.

Absorption of iron: Absorption of iron takes place mainly in the upper portion of the small intestine. Most of the iron enters the bloodstream directly and not through the lymphatics. The precise mechanism by which this absorption takes place across the mucosal cells is not known. Evidence indicates that absorption is regulated to some extent by physiological demand. The important factors may be iron stores, hypoxia, erythropoietic activity, and level of unsaturated iron-binding protein. Thus, persons who are iron-deficient tend to absorb iron more efficiently and in greater quantities than do normal subjects. This phenomenon has been demonstrated with medicinal ferrous sulfate and with food tagged with the radioactive isotope ^{59}Fe.

Several other factors affect iron absorption.[45] For example, phosphates and phytates in food reduce iron absorption, whereas ascorbic acid increases it. Malabsorption syndromes and gastrectomy reduce absorption, whereas pyridoxine deficiency, untreated pernicious anemia, and chronic pancreatic insufficiency increase the absorption of iron. Studies have indicated that egg yolk, despite its relatively large amount of iron, inhibits the absorption of iron not only in the yolk but also in other foods.

The availability of iron from foodstuffs varies greatly. Healthy subjects normally absorb only 5% to 10% of the iron in their foods, whereas iron-deficient subjects may absorb twice that amount. Therefore, if a diet were to supply 15 mg of iron, the normal person would absorb 0.75 to 1.5 mg of iron but the iron-deficient person would absorb as much as 3 mg. Similarly, absorption is generally increased during growth and pregnancy, after bleeding, and in other conditions in which the demand for iron is enhanced.

Requirements: From the above it is clear that dietary requirements of iron are approximately ten times the body's physiological requirements. If a normally healthy man or postmenopausal woman requires 1 mg of iron daily because of iron losses, then the dietary requirements are about 10 mg per day. This allows a fair margin of safety, as absorption is increased with need.

Menstrual loss of iron has been estimated to average a little under 1 mg per day during an entire year.[46] It is recommended that women of childbearing age have a dietary intake of 18 mg per day.

The average daily iron requirement necessary to develop the fetus and supportive tissues and to expand the maternal blood supply during pregnancy is about 1.5 mg. Most of this additional iron is required in the second and third trimesters of pregnancy.

No satisfactory studies have yet established iron requirements or rate of iron absorption during lactation. Human breast milk contains about 0.2 mg iron/dl, so a woman in full lactation might be losing 1 mg or more of iron per day.

Infants are born with stores of iron that are adequate for the first three months of life. Premature infants may have reduced iron stores at birth and are therefore more liable to develop iron-deficiency anemia. Recommended Dietary Allowances (RDA)* of iron range from 10 mg (for infants 1 month old) to 15 mg (for children 1 to 3 years old).

Deficiency: A glance at the nutritional requirements for iron and the iron content of commonly eaten foods might suggest that iron deficiency is rare, but such is not the case. Food iron is poorly absorbed. Iron is not readily excreted into the urine or into the gastrointestinal tract, and severe iron deficiency is usually associated with an increased need for iron that results from conditions such as pregnancy, blood loss, or expansion of the total body mass during growth. Iron deficiency is most common in young children, in women during the childbearing age, and in persons with chronic blood loss.

*See page 12

Many people may be unaware or unconcerned about chronic blood loss that occurs, for example, in mild peptic ulcer, bleeding gums, hemorrhoids, menorrhagia, and tropical parasitic diseases such as hookworm infestation or schistosomiasis. Whenever blood is lost, iron is lost, and if not replaced it will eventually lead to iron-deficiency anemia (see anemias, page 26).

In addition to its well-known role in erythrocyte formation, iron may play a role in host resistance to infection. In that regard, iron deficiency evidently has a double deleterious effect: (1) by decreasing the activity of myeloperoxidase, a granulocytic enzyme that helps to destroy ingested bacteria, and (2) by decreasing the immune response.

Excess: Hemosiderosis is a condition in which, for any of a number of causes, the body has accumulated excessive stores of iron. These causes have included frequent blood transfusions, especially for hemolytic anemia (in this condition the erythrocytes are destroyed but their iron is not lost to the body), excessive oral or parenteral doses of therapeutic iron, and excessive consumption of iron in food. For example, the diet of the Bantu natives of South Africa contains quantities of iron often exceeding 100 mg per day – the result of using iron utensils in their daily cooking and for the preparation of fermented beverages.[47] Excessive accumulation of iron is also seen in hemochromatosis, a disease believed to be due to an inborn error of metabolism in which excessive iron is absorbed from the diet. The danger of excessive ingestion of medicinal iron is constantly present, especially as enthusiastic advertising leads the health-conscious layman to believe that iron is a body strengthener and a tonic. This may result in persons believing that the more that is taken, the better for their health. A large variety of iron-containing medicinal preparations are available without prescription. As a result, it is common for some persons to be consuming many times the daily recommended allowances for iron. Accidental poisoning with ferrous sulfate has sometimes been fatal in children.

In iron overload, the plasma iron content is high, the iron binding capacity is depressed, and the percent saturation is nearly complete. Iron overload is unknown from iron fortification of foods.

Calcium and Phosphorus

Although calcium and phosphorus are not chemically related, they occur together in the body in a ratio that is nearly constant. About 1.5% of the human body is composed of calcium and about 1% is composed of phosphorus. These two minerals are present mainly in the bones, where the calcium combines with phosphorus as various calcium phosphate salts to form a hard substance that gives the body rigidity. However, the skeleton of the body is not the rigid unchanging structure it appears to be. In fact, the bones contain a cellular matrix, and calcium is continuously taken up by the bones and given back to the body. The bones also function as a reservoir for these minerals. Appreciable loss or gain in calcium is usually reflected in similar changes in phosphorus content.

Calcium

The body of a healthy adult contains about 1250 gm of calcium, 99% of which is in the bones and teeth. Calcium is present in the blood serum in small but important quantities, usually about 10 mg/dl of serum. A substantial reduction in this amount causes the development of tetany, whereas an increase may lead to respiratory or cardiac failure due to impaired muscle function. Approximately 60% of serum calcium is ionized and the remainder is bound to serum proteins. The extracellular fluids and soft tissues of an adult contain approximately 10 gm of calcium.

Sources: A great variety of foods such as whole-grain cereal products, leafy vegetables, legumes, and nuts contain calcium; particularly rich sources are milk and cheese. Sardines and other small fish whose bones are eaten are other important sources of calcium. Cow's milk contains 120 mg/dl, considerably more than human milk (30 mg/dl).

Ordinarily, meat is low in calcium and fluoride, but mechanically deboned meat (because of the way it is processed) contains finely ground bone particles and therefore does serve as an extra source of those nutrients. Mechanically deboned meat will probably become an important addition to our meat supply as our society becomes more resourceful and less wasteful.

Absorption: Calcium absorption depends on several factors, but vitamin D is one of the most important. Thus, even if the intake of calcium is adequate, calcium absorption is reduced and calcium balance may be negative if the subject is deficient in vitamin D.

Certain amino acids, citric acid, and lactose enhance calcium absorption. In contrast, phosphates, phytates, and oxalates inhibit calcium absorption. It is doubtful, however, if any of these substances are ordinarily important determinants of the calcium requirements of man.

Of considerable importance in calcium metabolism and calcium requirements is the human power of adaptation. The physical basis of adaptation is not proved but its existence is clear.

Persons who eat low-calcium diets have been shown to absorb calcium more efficiently than do those who customarily eat foods higher in calcium. Thus, as the intake of calcium is lowered, the efficiency of the body to absorb and retain calcium increases; the calcium intake results in reduced utilization.

Calcium is present in the feces, urine, and sweat. In the feces, the calcium is primarily of dietary origin which for a number of reasons has not been absorbed. The amount of calcium in the urine varies greatly but usually is that which has been absorbed but not taken up by the skeleton or soft tissues. Persons who work in high temperatures may lose considerable quantities of calcium in sweat.

Requirements: The specific human requirement for calcium is difficult to determine because of the "adaptation mechanism," the many other factors influencing absorption, and the variability in calcium loss from the body. The RDA, 800 mg daily for adults, is well above theoretical estimates of need.

The FAO/WHO Expert Group[48] suggested that a practical allowance for adults would be an intake of 400 to 500 mg daily.

Additional calcium is needed during pregnancy and lactation. The fetus has its calcium needs, and human milk contains 30 mg of calcium per dl. An extra 400 mg of calcium above the normal adult recommendation is suggested for pregnant women and for lactating women. Without this the woman is likely to deplete her own calcium reserves. This extra calcium is readily supplied by an extra pint of milk.

The skeletons of children are constantly increasing in size, so they have especially high calcium requirements. The Recommended Dietary Allowance is 500 mg for infants (which incidentally is higher than the amount that would be obtained from breast milk), increasing to 1200 mg daily during the pubertal growth spurt and the teenage period.

Deficiency: Despite the publicity given to the importance of a high calcium intake and the scientific work done on calcium requirements in adult man, there is no convincing evidence to show that a low intake of calcium even at levels of 250 to 300 mg daily is harmful. Presumably, adults achieve balance at the level of intake supplied by their usual diet, largely because of "adaptation."

In females on a habitually low calcium intake, depletion of body calcium resulting from repeated pregnancies and prolonged lactation may play a role in the development of osteomalacia. However, vitamin D deficiency is far more often implicated in this condition.

Even in children, the development of rickets is known to be largely independent of calcium intake. There is still no convincing evidence to determine whether low calcium intakes, so commonly found in developing countries, adversely affect the growth of children.

Osteoporosis is a common disease of aging in the United States and in many other parts of the world. Loss of bone may be an inevitable process of aging and usually starts in middle age. Although high-calcium diets are frequently recommended in osteoporosis and in the diets of the elderly, there is no good scientific evidence to show that this measure actually increases bone density. There is now evidence to show that a high intake of fluoride benefits calcium retention and lessens osteoporosis.

Excess: Certain populations, such as the Masai in East Africa, whose diets consist almost exclusively of milk, may have intakes of over 2000 mg calcium per day. This has not been shown to have any deleterious effects.

However, there are conditions in which excessive calcium is found in the serum, urine, or soft tissues – conditions such as idiopathic hypercalcemia, the "milk-alkali syndrome," renal-stone formation, hypercalciuria, and fluorosis. There are no current epidemiologic data to prove that high calcium intakes are responsible for these conditions.

Iodide

The body of an average adult contains about 40 mg of iodide, of which about half is present in the thyroid gland. Iodide is essential for the formation of thyroxine and triiodothyronine, the hormones of the thyroid.

Sources: Iodide is present in rocks and soils, but through the ages much has been washed into the sea. Man gets his iodide from food and from water, the iodide content of which varies according to the iodide content of their source. Thus there are waters with a fairly high content of iodide and others with negligible amounts, and the same foodstuffs grown in different soils have different iodide contents.

Seafoods on the whole are rich in iodide; dairy products, eggs, and some vegetables may also be good sources. Iodized salt is sold in the United States, but people often don't know

58

Figure 31. **Figure 31.** Missing teeth per adult (fluoride and nonfluoride communities).

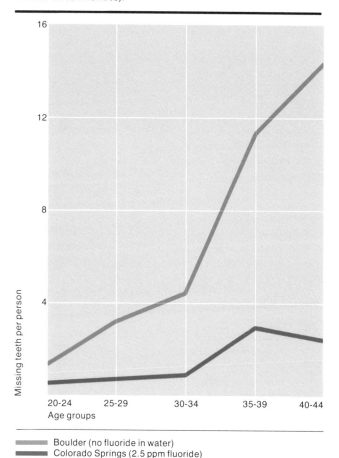

Boulder (no fluoride in water)
Colorado Springs (2.5 ppm fluoride)

That the benefits of fluoride accrued during childhood are carried over into adulthood is shown by a comparison of missing teeth of adults in Boulder, Colorado (no fluoride in the drinking water) and Colorado Springs (2.5 ppm of fluoride in the drinking water). At age 40-44 the loss of teeth is less than 4 permanent teeth per person in Colorado Springs while it averages about 16 permanent teeth loss per person in Boulder, Colorado. The ratio of tooth loss is 4 to 5 times greater, at all times, in the nonfluoride area than in the fluoride area from age 20 to 44.

whether they are buying iodized or noniodized salt, and even institutions such as hospitals and schools are frequently found to be using noniodized salt – a most unfortunate situation. Most salt in processed foods is noniodized, because iodized salt leads to technical problems in processing.

The Food and Nutrition Board of our National Research Council has recommended federal legislation mandating the iodization of all salt marketed for human consumption. However, there is as yet no federal legislation concerning salt, and state laws are not uniform. A suitable iodide level is 0.5 gm potassium iodide per 1 kg of purified salt.

Although the consumption of iodized salt has apparently decreased in recent years, it is not at all clear that total iodide intake has decreased. New dough conditioners in bakeries evidently provide considerable amounts of iodide, and milk and dyes may well supply further iodide. Indeed, decreases in radio-iodide uptake by the thyroid observed in recent years suggest that iodide consumption in the United States is actually increasing.

Absorption and utilization: In normal people, iodide is readily absorbed from the intestinal tract, and about one third is utilized by the thyroid gland while two thirds is excreted in the urine. Iodide nutriture can be studied by determining the avidity of the thyroid gland to take up radioactive iodide, by measurement of the stable iodide content of the urine and by determination of the protein-bound iodide. Iodide in the feces comes mainly from the bile.

Requirements: It has been suggested that 1 μg of iodide per kg body weight is an adequate intake in the human. However, growing children and women during pregnancy and lactation have increased needs.

Deficiency: A deficiency of iodide leads to the development of goiter, but there are several other causes of goiter besides iodide deficiency. Endemic goiter (see page 46) occurs where population groups have dietary sources of iodide below normal requirements. In many parts of the world (but less so in the United States), iodide deficiency is a significant public health problem[49] because we do not consistently use iodized salt.

Iodide-deficiency goiter is really a defense mechanism designed to keep thyroid hormones at an optimal level. A decrease in the circulating concentrations of iodide-containing thyroid hormones triggers a release of thyroid-stimulating hormone (TSH) from the pituitary gland. This eventually causes thyroid hypertrophy and an increase in the number of thyroid epithelial cells.

Goitrogens in brassica plants such as cabbage have been shown to increase the needs for iodide in certain laboratory animals. As a result, iodide intakes that would be adequate under normal circumstances failed to prevent goiter in animals that consumed large quantities of goitrogens. There is little evidence to show that goitrogens in normal diets have been important in the production of goiter in man, although recent studies in Colombia raise the possibility.[50]

Fluoride

In human beings, fluoride deposition is found mainly in the teeth and the skeleton but the total quantity is small. However, the presence of traces of this mineral in the teeth helps to protect them against caries and, as such, fluoride is essential to optimal health and is thus referred to as a mineral nutrient.

The protective effect of fluoride occurs primarily during infancy and early childhood when the teeth are developing, but its caries-preventive action is carried over into adulthood as long as one has access to fluoridated water (Figure 31). Studies suggest that fluoride has a second role in strengthening bone and that an adequate fluoride intake is important as a protection against osteoporosis.[51]

Recent studies show that fluoride is also necessary for growth in rats and fertility in mice.[52]

Sources: Most foods contain traces of fluoride, but not enough to be effective in reducing dental decay.

The main source of fluoride for humans is the water they drink. If water contains about 1 part per million (ppm) of fluoride, it will supply adequate amounts of this mineral nutrient. Many waters contain quantities of fluoride much less than that, and the addition of fluoride (fluoridation) to raise its level in water to what is considered optimal is an important public health measure. Fluoridation has been shown to reduce the incidence of dental caries by 60% to 70%.

Requirements: An intake of about 1 to 2 mg per day is considered adequate. A water supply containing 1 part per million of fluoride will supply 1 to 2 mg per day, depending on the consumption of water and other beverages made with that water, such as coffee, tea, soft drinks, and those reconstituted from frozen fruit drinks.

Deficiency: A deficiency of fluoride during infancy and childhood leaves the teeth relatively unprotected from dental caries. Tooth decay is a major public health problem that has important economic implications. Increasing evidence indicates that there is less osteoporosis in areas where the fluoride

content of the water is high than in comparable areas where the fluoride content of the water is low. There are good data to show that osteoporosis improves if large doses of fluoride are administered therapeutically. Recent evidence suggests that arterial calcification may be less marked in high-fluoride than in low-fluoride areas.[15]

Excess: An excessively high intake of fluoride during childhood causes a condition known as dental fluorosis, in which the teeth become mottled and somewhat discolored (Figures 32 and 33). Very large intakes of fluoride cause bone changes with increased bone density, calcification of muscle insertions, and exostoses. The condition can be diagnosed most easily by radiographic means. The most likely places to find these changes is in roentgenograms of the forearm (Figure 34). Dental and skeletal fluorosis do not occur in communities with properly controlled fluoridated water supplies. Fluorosis is found in certain defined areas of India,[53] Tanzania,[54] the western parts of the United States, and other areas where the water sometimes contains 10 to 45 ppm of fluoride, well above the level of 1 ppm used in fluoridation. Fluorosis has occasionally occurred in industrial workers as the result of chronic intoxication due to prolonged contact with high concentrations of fluoride compounds used in certain manufacturing processes.

Sodium and Potassium

Sodium and potassium are essential elements in the human body. Sodium is present in greatest concentration in extracellular fluid. Its role is to maintain equilibrium between the extracellular and intracellular fluid compartments. The other functions of sodium include its role in maintaining the pH of blood, its involvement with potassium in muscle contractility, and its activity in the conduction of nerve impulses. Potassium, on the other hand, is the main cation of the cells, and its concentration in the intracellular fluid is greater than in the extracellular fluid.

Sources: Although foods of both animal and plant origin contain sodium, the former usually contain more. In American diets, most of the sodium usually comes from salt added at the table, cooked with the food, or added during processing. Bacon, ham, sausage, butter, and certain other foods are salted during preparation, and foods such as bread have salt added. Man has added salt to his food for more than 3,000 years, but in normal circumstances there appears to be no actual nutritional need for more sodium than is present in raw foods. An increasingly common source of sodium in our diets is

60

Figure 32. Dental caries and dental fluorosis in relation to fluoride in public water supplies.

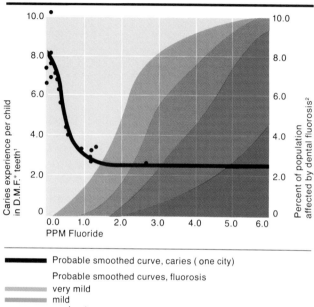

Probable smoothed curve, caries (one city)

Probable smoothed curves, fluorosis
- very mild
- mild
- moderate
- severe

1. Adapted from Dean HT: New York Symposium, 1945.
2. Adapted from Dean HT: *Int Dent J 4*:311-337, 1954.
*D.M.F. = Decayed, missing, and filled.

Figure 33. Moderate fluorosis shown as mottling of the permanent teeth. This 14-year-old drank well water containing 5.5 ppm of fluoride from birth (5.5 times optimum level).

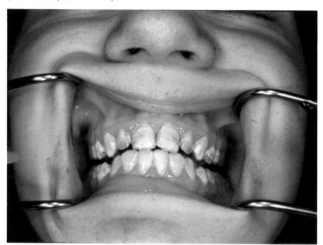

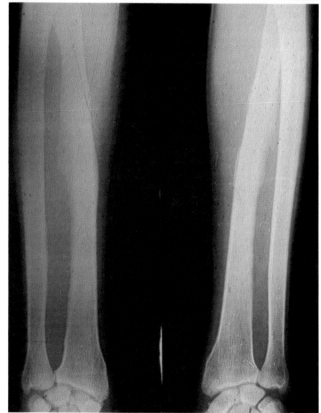

Figure 34. Skeletal fluorosis (18 times optimum level). This resulted from prolonged consumption of water from a stream containing 18 ppm of fluoride. X-ray of forearm shows calcific deposits between the radius and ulna.

monosodium glutamate, which is a flavor enhancer.

Potassium is ubiquitous and is present in most commonly eaten foods. A dietary deficiency of potassium does not occur in those who eat an ordinary mixed diet. Bananas, oranges, avocados, and some other foods are rich sources of potassium (see Appendix A).

Requirements: The Food and Nutrition Board has not established RDAs for sodium or potassium. Intakes of sodium in the United States average about 5 gm per day per person (equals about 13 gm of salt) – at least five times greater than physiological needs.

Intakes of potassium in the United States are usually between 0.8 and 1.5 gm per 1000 Calories consumed, with minimal needs believed to be between 0.8 and 1.3 gm per day.

Deficiency: Excessive and prolonged sweating from any cause may lead to symptoms and signs of salt depletion if only the water is replaced and not the lost salt. Giddiness, nausea, apathy, exhaustion, cramps (often termed "miner's cramps"), vomiting, and, finally, respiratory failure may result. When profuse sweating occurs, such symptoms can be prevented simply by adding a little more salt to food or, in extreme cases, by adding about 1 gm of salt per liter to the water consumed. Salt tablets are not necessary.

Sodium depletion may also result from severe vomiting and diarrhea, during adrenocortical failure, as a result of excessive use of diuretics, and in certain renal diseases.

Potassium deficiency is associated with general muscle weakness, which may lead to reduced intestinal tone and distention, to cardiac abnormalities, and to respiratory failure. Less severe but chronic depletion results in what is termed "hypokalemic nephropathy." Common causes of potassium depletion are the infectious and nutritional diarrheas of infancy,[55] which are often termed "weanling diarrheas." Care must be taken to ensure an adequate potassium intake in those on a restricted diet, those taking diuretics, and hospital patients receiving parenteral nourishment and intravenous fluids.

Excess: There is increasing interest in the possibility that our unnecessarily high intakes of dietary sodium (mostly from salt) may play a role in the etiology of hypertension in genetically predisposed persons.

The lethal effects of large intakes of sodium chloride are illustrated in several reports of infants having been accidentally fed a saline mixture in place of water, glucose, or some other fluid in a formula diet.

Magnesium

Magnesium is an essential constituent of all soft tissue and bone in man. It is an important metallic cation in living cells and is required in enzymes responsible for energy transformation of phosphate bonds. The adult body contains about 25 gm of magnesium, of which approximately 70% is found in the bones. The skeleton evidently provides the body's magnesium stores.

Sources: Most foods, especially those of vegetable origin, contain useful amounts of magnesium. Whole-grain cereal products, potatoes, vegetables, and fruits provide most of the magnesium in human diets.

Absorption: In contrast to calcium, vitamin D does not aid in magnesium absorption. Failure of absorption is not known to be a problem.

Requirements: The RDA of magnesium is 300 to 350 mg for normal adults, 450 mg for women who are pregnant or lactating, and 50 to 70 mg for infants.[3]

Deficiency: Magnesium deficiency in human beings[56] results in a condition similar to hypocalcemic tetany.[57] Sufferers, usually alcoholics,[58] have low serum magnesium levels, and the condition responds dramatically to magnesium administration. Magnesium deficiency with kwashiorkor has also been described.[59]

Experimentally induced magnesium deficiency in animals leads to soft-tissue calcification and, in animals fed high-cholesterol diets, results in increased atherosclerosis. The role of low intakes of magnesium on atherogenesis in man is unknown. Many American diets are marginal in their content of magnesium.

Copper

Copper, widely distributed in food, is an essential nutrient required for the formation of hemoglobin as well as for the production and survival of erythrocytes. Evidence that ill health due to a dietary deficiency of copper occurs in man is unverified.

In Wilson's disease, or hepatolenticular degeneration, there is accumulation of excessive copper in the tissues, probably due to a genetic absence of a liver enzyme. It is characterized by neurological degeneration and cirrhotic liver changes. A reduction in dietary copper by the use of chelating agents to bind free copper may be useful in treatment.

Sulfur

Sulfur, an element present in all protein material and, therefore, all living matter in the human, is present mainly in the two sulfur-containing amino acids, methionine and cystine, plus the vitamins thiamin and biotin. Additionally, cells containing sulfate ions and free sulfhydryl (SH) groups are important in some enzyme systems. Sulfur is also present in chondroitin sulfate found in cartilage and bone.

It is likely that most of the required sulfur is obtained from dietary methionine and cystine, but some foods, notably onions, are rich in organic sulfur. Little is known of sulfur requirements or sulfur deficiency in man.

Zinc

It has been clearly established that zinc is an essential nutrient. Zinc is present in many enzyme systems, including carbonic anhydrase, the enzyme responsible for the formation of bicarbonate ions from carbon dioxide in the erythrocytes, stomach, pancreas, and kidney. Severe zinc deficiency has been identified in Iran and in Egypt, where it was found to be associated with hypogonadism and severe growth failure. Both conditions improved upon the administration of zinc. Investigators in Denver, Colorado, have reported on marginal zinc deficiences; how widespread or serious such deficiency is cannot at present be judged, but it is thought to be minimal. Zinc deficiency in animals leads to pathological changes in the skin; in human beings, zinc deficiency is said to be associated with ulcers, burns, and impaired healing of wounds. Zinc deficiency has recently been linked to acrodermatitis enteropathica, a rare inherited disease (usually fatal) with cutaneous manifestations similar to those of zinc deficiency in animals. Such patients have low plasma zinc concentrations; their condition typically improves when their diets are supplemented with zinc.

Human zinc requirements are not clearly known. The Food and Nutrition Board recommends 15 mg per day for adults, with daily supplements of 5 mg during pregnancy and 10 mg during lactation. Good sources are animal foods and whole grains. However, the increased amount of zinc in whole grains may be offset by its lesser availability resulting from binding to the fiber.

Chromium

For normal glucose metabolism, animals require trivalent chromium, which is a component of the so-called glucose tolerance factor (GTF). Investigations in the United States and abroad have suggested that some subjects have chromium-responsive disturbances of glucose metabolism. It is not clear what the clinical significance (if any) of these findings is. Furthermore, it has not yet proved possible to fix a chromium requirement. Good sources of chromium are animal foods, whole-grain products, and certain types of yeast.

Trace Elements

It is generally accepted that human beings require zinc, manganese, molybdenum, cobalt, selenium, and chromium. Bromide, tin, and vanadium may also be required but the evidence is vague. In fact, some scientists speculate that all elements may have some role in metabolism.

Much work details the important effects of experimentally induced deficiencies of these elements in animals, and there is little doubt that the same elements are also essential to man. Evidence suggests that some effects of deficiency may be found in severe malnutrition, particularly in kwashiorkor, in which the diet is deficient in protein, calories, and often many other nutrients.

These trace elements are all supplied in adequate quantities in normal diets; chances of deficiency are therefore very slight.

Vegetables (notably green leafy vegetables), cereals (especially if not highly refined), liver and kidney, seafood, and meat are good sources of most trace elements.

VITAMINS

Vitamins are organic substances — not carbohydrate, fat, or protein — that are present in minute quantities in foodstuffs and necessary for metabolism. They are classified together not because they are chemically related or because they have similar physiological functions, but more because of the way in which they were discovered and because in very small amounts they are vital factors in the diet and yet do not fit into the other categories of nutrients.

Vitamin A

History: Vitamin A is fat soluble. It was discovered about 60 years ago when scientists found that if the only form of fat in the diet of certain laboratory animals was pork lard, the animals ceased growing, whereas on an otherwise identical diet in which butter replaced the lard the animals grew and thrived. Clearly, butter contained some substance that was not present in lard. The substance seemed to be necessary for the health of the animals even though both diets contained adequate quantities of carbohydrates, fats, proteins, and minerals. Further experiments with animals showed that egg yolk and cod liver oil contained the same vital food factor, which was then named vitamin A.

A little later it was established that many vegetable products have the same nutritional properties as the vitamin A that is present in butter and other animal fats. Those plants were found to contain a yellow pigment, called carotene, which is converted to vitamin A in the human body.

Properties: Vitamin A is soluble in fat but insoluble in water. It is an almost colorless substance and is found only in foods of animal origin.

Carotenes occur widely in plants. In some foodstuffs, the yellow color of the carotenes is masked by the green color of chlorophyll, which often is present in close association with it. Several different carotenes act as provitamins, or precursors, of vitamin A. The conversion of these substances into vitamin A takes place mainly in the walls of the intestines but also in the liver and kidney.

The liver acts as the main store of vitamin A in the human and most of the vertebrates, hence the high concentration of this vitamin in fish liver oils.

Vitamin A has several known functions in the human body. Vitamin A aldehyde combines with opsin in scotopic vision. The vitamin participates in the synthesis of mucopolysaccharides and in the release of a protease that affects dissolution of the cartilaginous matrix. It also has a role in reproductive processes.

Units: Vitamin A activity is now measured in "retinol equivalents." By definition, one retinol equivalent is equal to one μg of retinol, or 6 μg of B-carotene, or 12 μg of other provitamin A carotinoids. International Units are no longer used, but since they are referred to in the older literature we will note that one retinol equivalent is equal to 3.33 IU of retinol or 10 IU of B-carotene.

Dietary Sources: Vitamin A itself is found only in animal products, and the main natural sources are butter, eggs, whole milk, liver, and some fish.

Many plant foods contain carotene. Good sources are dark-green leafy vegetables and various pigmented fruits and vegetables such as tomatoes, carrots, sweet potatoes, pumpkin, and papaya. Yellow corn is the only commonly eaten cereal that contains carotene. Red palm oil, which is produced and eaten in many tropical countries, is an extremely rich source.

In the United States, vitamin A is added to some foods such as margarine and dried milk powder, skimmed milk, and other low-fat milks.

Human requirements: The Food and Nutrition Board's RDA of vitamin A for adult males is 1000 retinol equivalents; for adult females the RDA is 800 retinol equivalents. For infants and children, the RDAs are somewhat more liberal to provide for growth and to ensure adequate body stores. For the second and third trimester of pregnancy an added daily allowance of 200 retinol equivalents and for lactation an added daily allowance of 400 retinol equivalents above that of the normal are recommended.

A number of factors affect absorption of provitamin A from the intestine. Carotene is poorly utilized in persons on a low-fat diet, and intestinal disease such as dysentery, celiac disease, and sprue limit the absorption of vitamin A and the conversion of carotene. Persons with obstruction of the bile ducts are likely to become deficient in vitamin A, because bile salts are essential for the absorption of vitamin A and carotene.

Tests of vitamin A status: Temporary lowering of vitamin A intake will have little effect on plasma vitamin A or carotene levels, because of large stores in the liver. Prolonged low intakes, however, will lead to lowering of the serum level, and in fact serum levels do correlate with dietary intake (Figure 35).[60] For adults, plasma retinol levels below 10 μg/dl are considered low (ie, indicate a high risk), 10 to 19 μg/dl are considered low (ie, indicate a moderate risk), and levels of 20 μg/dl or more are considered acceptable. For plasma carotene, the cutoff points are double those of retinol.[61]

Deficiency: A dietary deficiency of vitamin A[62] may result in the development of xerophthalmia, which may then lead to keratomalacia and blindness. This is a serious public health problem in some parts of the world (see page 35).

Early signs of vitamin A deficiency are night blindness and the development of dermatological lesions such as follicular hyperdermatosis and "crazy-pavement" skin. Another sign of vitamin A deficiency, though of limited diagnostic value, is Bitot spots, which occur bilaterally in the eyes and are seen as foamy patches on the lateral side of the cornea (see Figure 17).

Toxicity: Hypervitaminosis of vitamin A due to excessive intake has occurred with overmedication of vitamin preparations, in faddists who include extra-large doses of the vitamin in their diets, and in other circumstances in which excessive amounts are taken over long periods of time.

64

Figure 35. Relationship between average serum retinol levels and average daily intake of vitamin A activity in adult males in 11 countries surveyed by ICNND.

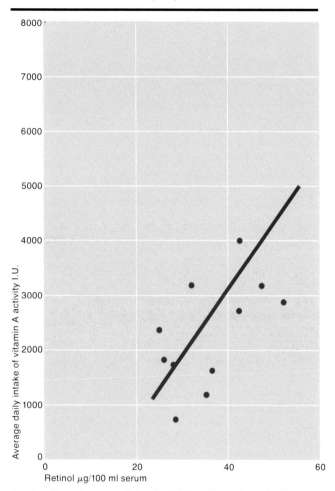

Adapted with permission from: Patwardhan VN: Hypovitaminosis A and epidemiology of xerophthalmia. *Amer J Clin Nutr 22*:1106, 1969.

The signs and symptoms include lethargy, malaise, abdominal pain, headaches, excessive sweating, and brittle nails. Carotenoid deposits may cause a yellow dyspigmentation of the soles of the feet, the palms of the hands, and the nasolabial folds. Increased intracranial pressure and edema may develop.

Acute toxicity has been observed in Arctic explorers who consumed large amounts of polar bear liver, an organ unusually rich in vitamin A (up to 600,000 retinol equivalents per 100 gm of liver). Toxicity has also been observed in children given single massive doses of vitamin A.

Thiamin (Vitamin B₁)

History: The tale of Eijkman and his chickens (like the story of Jenner and his cow vaccine) is a classic example of how an astute observation in an unlikely place led to a historical landmark in the advancement of science. Working in Batavia, Java (now Djakarta, Indonesia), this Dutch physician noted that hens fed a diet of leftover rice cooked for human consumption developed a disease like beriberi. When fed either whole-grain rice or rice polishings, they recovered.[63] Eijkman believed that the polished rice contained a toxin that could be neutralized by something in rice polishings, and he published his findings in 1897. In 1901, Grijns first postulated that beriberi might be due to something lacking in polished rice.[64] In 1916, McCollum and Kennedy reported finding a water-soluble B vitamin that they believed to be the antiberiberi factor.[65] The vitamin was subsequently divided into its antiberiberi and antipellagra factors. Finally, vitamin B₁, subsequently to be called thiamin, was isolated and then synthesized.

Properties: Thiamin hydrochloride is a compound consisting of a pyrimidine ring joined by a methylene bridge to a thiazole nucleus. The bond between the two rings is weak, with the result that the compound is easily destroyed in an alkaline medium. Thiamin is highly soluble in water and will resist temperatures up to 100°C but tends to be destroyed with more heat. That fact has practical implications; the vitamin is destroyed in food fried in a hot pan or cooked too long under pressure. Because of its solubility, thiamin is easily leached out of foodstuffs being washed or boiled.

Malnourished alcoholics have a decreased ability to absorb thiamin, a phenomenon evidently related to folate nutrition, inasmuch as folate-depleted rats do not absorb thiamin well.

Thiamin pyrophosphate functions in carbohydrate metabolism as a coenzyme in the decarboxylation of alpha-keto acids and in transketolase. Without cocarboxylase, pyruvic acid accumulates in various tissues, and pyruvic acid accumulation tends to occur in thiamin deficiency. A specific relationship between thiamin nutrition and transketolase activity at the enzyme or cellular level has likewise been observed in man.[66]

Thiamin is easily absorbed from the intestinal tract, but the body is unable to store any quantity of thiamin. The liver, heart, and brain have a higher concentration than muscle tissue or other organs. A person on a high-thiamin intake soon becomes saturated and begins to excrete increased quantities in the urine.

Units: The activity of thiamin hydrochloride is expressed in mg of the chemically pure synthesized substance.

Dietary sources: Thiamin is found in foods of both animal and vegetable origin. The richest sources among commonly eaten foods are pork, whole-grain and enriched cereals, and the seeds of legumes. Green vegetables, fish, meat, fruit, and milk all contain useful quantities.

In cereals, thiamin is present mainly in the germ and outer coat of the seed, and much of the vitamin is lost if cereals are milled and refined.

Several antithiamins have been described. Two are thermolabile, and they catalyze the breakdown of thiamin. The first, thiaminase I, is found in the viscera of fresh-water fish and in microorganisms, whereas thiaminase II is found only in microorganisms. Thermostable thiamin antagonists have been found in plants and animal tissues.[67]

Human requirements: The Recommended Daily Allowance for thiamin is 0.4 mg per 1000 Calories for all ages, with an added allowance of 0.4 mg daily during the second and third trimester of pregnancy and 0.5 mg daily during lactation. For those older adults who consume less than 2000 Calories daily, 1.0 mg of thiamin daily is recommended.

Tests of thiamin status: The classical test of thiamin status has been thiamin excretion in the urine, expressed as μgm/thiamin/gm of creatinine, and guidelines for its interpretation are given by Sauberlich et al.[61] Since the work of Brin,[66] however, the effect of added thiamin pyrophosphate on erythrocyte transketolase activity has been used in testing. Hemolyzed whole blood is incubated with excess ribose-5-phosphate, and the activity (loss of ribose-5-phosphate or production of end products) is measured. In a similar procedure, thiamin pyrophosphate is added, and the increased activity (expressed as a percentage of the baseline activity) is the measured effect. Sauberlich et al described an effect of less than 15% as accept-

able, one from 16% to 20% as indicative of medium risk, and one greater than 20% as indicative of high risk.

Deficiency: A deficiency of thiamin is the cause of the disease beriberi. Beriberi occurs mainly among rice-eating peoples and is common in Asia. In the United States, thiamin deficiency is fairly common among alcoholics (Figure 36) and may lead to Wernicke's disease and Korsakoff's syndrome (see page 39).

Toxicity: When thiamin is taken in excessive amounts, it is excreted in the urine and hence has no known toxicity. The kidney has no known threshold.

Riboflavin

History: Early work on the properties of vitamins in yeast and other foodstuffs showed that the antineuritic factors were destroyed by heat but that a growth-promoting factor was not destroyed. This heat-stable vitamin was finally isolated from milk, and the yellow crystals were named riboflavin. In 1935 it was synthesized by the German chemist Kuhn, who had also been responsible for its isolation.

Properties: Riboflavin functions as a coenzyme or active prosthetic group of flavoproteins concerned with tissue oxidation and respiration. The vitamin plays an important role in both protein and energy metabolism. Riboflavin is a water-soluble, yellow, crystalline substance. It is heat stable in an acid solution but decomposes in an alkaline solution or on exposure to sunlight.

Experimentally induced riboflavin deficiency in animals causes a failure of growth as well as lesions of the skin and eyes.

Units: Riboflavin is measured in mg of the chemically pure substance.

Dietary sources: Many foods of animal and vegetable origin contain riboflavin. The richest sources are milk and its nonfat products. Other good sources are green vegetables, meat (especially liver), fish, and eggs. A portion of the riboflavin is lost when food is cooked or exposed to sunlight or if the water in which the food is cooked is discarded. Milk in bottles exposed to direct sunlight loses some of its riboflavin content.

Human requirements: In the United States, the RDAs for riboflavin are 1.7 mg for men and 1.3 mg for women. An additional 0.3 mg is recommended for women during the last two thirds of pregnancy and an additional 0.5 mg during lactation. Children have relatively higher needs than adults; RDAs range from 0.4 mg during infancy to 1.7 mg for adolescent boys.

Figure 36A. Beriberi heart. This patient was a chronic alcoholic whose diet had been poor for a long time; polyneuritis and congestive heart failure accompanied cardiac dilation. Thiamine deficiency leads to impaired function and enlargement of the heart, particularly of the right auricle and ventricle, shown by X-ray.

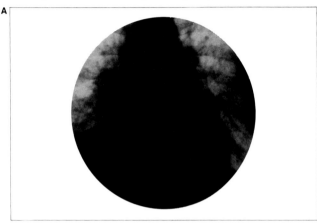

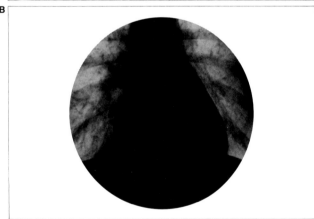

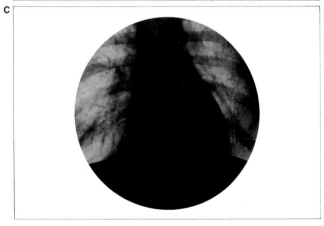

Figure 36B. After 1 week of thiamine therapy.

Figure 36C. After 3 weeks' treatment, progressive reduction in heart size is visible.

These allowances provide what is considered a reasonable margin of safety. The minimum requirement to prevent clinical signs of deficiency in adults is believed to be about 0.3 mg/1000 calories.

Tests of riboflavin status: As with tests for most water-soluble vitamins, the initial test for riboflavin status was based on riboflavin excretion in μg/gm of creatinine. A guide to the interpretation of such values is given by Sauberlich et al.

Riboflavin status is usually assessed by measuring the activation of erythrocyte glutathione reductase (EGR) by flavine adenine dinucleotide (FAD). Although the reduction uses nicotinamide coenzymes, the enzyme is a flavin enzyme with FAD as a prosthetic group, and it was found that enzyme activity decreased in riboflavin-depleted rats and humans. The addition of FAD to the incubation mixture led to little or no change in activity in subjects on a diet that included riboflavin, but in subjects on a low-riboflavin diet it led to a considerable increase in activity. This effect is expressed as an activity coefficient, which is the ratio of the amount of glutathione reduced with added FAD to the amount reduced without added FAD. If it is less than 1.2, it is considered acceptable; if 1.2 to 1.4, it indicates medium risk; and if greater than 1.4, it indicates high risk.

Deficiency: Naturally occurring riboflavin deficiency alone has not been shown to cause serious life-threatening disease in man. Ariboflavinosis does, however, lead to lesions of the lips, mouth, eyes, skin, and genitalia.[68]

The most-common lesions are angular stomatitis and cheilosis. Angular stomatitis consists of fissures or cracks radiating from the angles of the mouth onto the skin (Figures 37 and 38). Sometimes the lesions extend onto the mucous membrane inside the mouth. These cracks have a raw appearance but may become yellowish as a result of secondary infection. Cheilosis is a condition in which there are painful cracks on the upper and lower lips. The lips may be swollen and denuded at the line of closure. The lesions may be red and sore or dry and healing.

Less commonly, glossitis develops and causes a patchy denudation, papillary atrophy, and so-called magenta tongue. These latter conditions are not exclusively due to riboflavin deficiency.

Scrotal dermatitis in males (Figure 39) and vulval dermatitis in females have been particularly well described in experimentally induced riboflavin deficiency. The affected skin is usually intensely itchy and tends to desquamate. The

Figure 37A. Riboflavin deficiency manifested as fissures at angle of mouth.

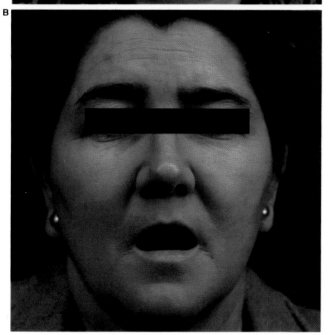

Induced riboflavin deficiency. Twelve of 15 male patients maintained for 9-17 months on a riboflavin-deficient but otherwise adequate diet (0.55 mg riboflavin daily per 2,200 calories) displayed clinical signs of deficiency including angular stomatitis, seborrheic dermatitis, and scaly scrotal skin lesions. Three of the four controls who were on the vitamin-deficient diet supplemented with 2 mg riboflavin daily, developed scrotal erythema with little or no scaling.

Figure 38. Angular stomatitis with bilateral fissures. Left oral lesion began after about 4½ months on the deficient diet and continued in a fluctuating state of exacerbation and remission for several months. Right lesion appeared 6 weeks after one at left with no preceding infection, and healed in about three weeks without recurrence.

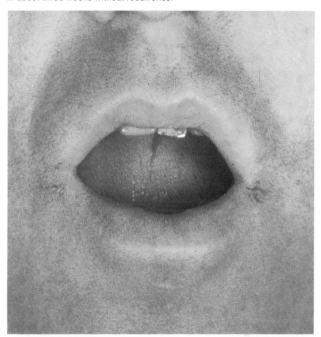

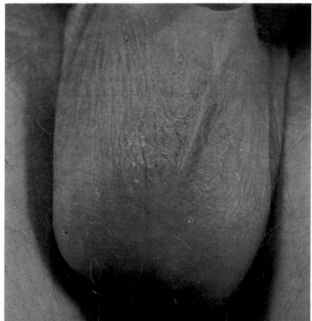

Figure 37B. Complete healing after treatment with riboflavin.

Figure 39. One patient developed scaly pruritic dermatitis on an erythematous base involving only the anterior aspect of the scrotum bilaterally. Other developments were patchy seborrhea of the scalp and vertical fissures around the nostrils (following a respiratory infection) that progressed to a weeping, crusty lesion. All were resistant to treatment. With 6 mg of riboflavin added to the diet, improvement of the scrotal lesion was prompt and unequivocal; healing of the more chronic lesions was slower but also definite.

68

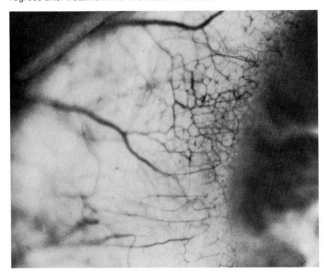

Figure 40. Beginning vascularization of the cornea. Vessels of the limbic plexus have proliferated and invaded the cornea. Vascularization may be accompanied by itching, burning, a feeling of grittiness in the eyes, and photophobia. All symptoms and signs regress after treatment with the vitamin riboflavin.

resulting scratching leads to redness, excoriation, and sometimes infection.

Eye lesions, again not specific to riboflavin deficiency, include vascularization of the cornea, photophobia, and lacrimation (Figures 40 and 41). The condition may cause an annoying irritation of the eyes, with itching and burning.

Dyssebacea, which is seen most commonly in the nasolabial folds but may involve the nose, the canthi of the eyes, and occasionally the ears, is a feature of riboflavin deficiency and certain other conditions. With a magnifying glass, one can see plugs of yellowish keratin standing out from the ducts of enlarged sebaceous glands.

Toxicity: Excess intake of riboflavin spills into the urine. Toxicity in man has not been reported.

Niacin (Nicotinic Acid)

History: Just as the history of thiamin is linked with the disease beriberi, so the history of niacin is inextricably woven with the story of the disease pellagra. Beriberi is associated with the New World and corn (maize)-eating peoples.

Well over 200 years ago Casal attributed pellagra to a poor diet, yet not until this century was the missing nutrient described and isolated. Investigators had been confused, partly because the disease pellagra could be cured by a protein-rich diet and was thought therefore to be due to a protein deficiency. Later, a liver extract almost devoid of protein was shown to cure pellagra, and in 1926 Goldberger demonstrated that yeast extract contains a nonprotein pellagra-preventing substance. In 1937, Elvehjem isolated niacinamide (nicotinic acid amide), which was found to cure "black tongue," a pellagra-like disease in dogs.

Properties: Niacin functions in the body as a component of two coenzymes important in glycolysis and tissue respiration. It is a simple derivative of pyridine and is extremely stable. Niacin is a water-soluble white compound that is moderately resistant to heat and to both acid and alkaline solutions. It is related chemically to nicotine but has very different physiological properties and is essentially nontoxic. Niacin (but not niacinamide) in very large oral doses will lower serum cholesterol (beta-lipoproteins and triglycerides) concentrations in man.

Niacin has been accepted in the United States as the name for nicotinic acid, and niacinamide for nicotinic acid amide.

Units: Niacin is measured in mg of the synthesized pure substance.

Figure 41A. Generalized dermatitis and growth failure in riboflavin-deficient rat. There is marked keratitis of the cornea.

Figure 41A. Generalized dermatitis and growth failure in riboflavin-deficient rat. There is marked keratitis of the cornea.

Figure 41B. After one month of treatment with riboflavin the animal shows improvement. Growth has been resumed and ocular and skin lesions are practically gone.

Figure 41C. After two months of treatment the rat shows no signs of the original deficiency.

Dietary sources: Niacin is present in many foods of vegetable origin, and niacinamide is present in most foods from animal sources. Particularly rich are lean meat (especially liver), peanuts, yeast, and cereal bran or germ. Beans, peas, and other legumes are good sources, but starch roots such as potatoes and cassava (manioc, yucca), common vegetables and fruits, and milk are all poor sources of the vitamin. Like other B vitamins, the main source in the diet is frequently the cereal staple consumed. Whole-grain or lightly milled cereals contain more niacin than do refined cereal grains and flours. Accumulating evidence suggests that part of the niacin in certain foodstuffs, especially cereals, is not available. Presumably, it is bound in a nonusable form.[69] Niacin is now often added to many manufactured food products, especially those made from cereals.

The human body has the ability to convert the amino acid tryptophan to niacin. It is believed that about 60 mg of dietary tryptophan is equivalent to 1 mg of niacin. Diets in the United States often contain 600 mg or more of tryptophan, which provides a substantial contribution to the niacin pool. However, diets of poor persons in the United States and elsewhere are usually low in protein, and pellagra is likely to occur among the poor. The tryptophan content of their diets is often as low as 150 mg.

Corn is poor in niacin, and its principal protein, zein, is very low in tryptophan content. There is evidence that some of the niacin in corn is present in a bound form and may be unavailable.

The results of studies in India suggest that there is more to pellagra than a simple deficiency of niacin plus tryptophan.[70] Millet contains adequate amounts of niacin and is not poor in tryptophan, but it is high in leucine. Black tongue developed in dogs that had been fed a diet composed of 65% millet. Adding leucine to a casein-based diet was also found to result in tryptophan-metabolism changes that were partially reversed by the addition of niacin. This seemed to suggest that pellagra in millet eaters might be partially caused by amino acid imbalance.

Human requirements: Because niacin is obtained either preformed or from tryptophan, the recommended allowances are stated as niacin equivalents. These include the preformed vitamin and the precursor tryptophan (60 mg tryptophan representing 1 mg niacin). RDAs in the United States are 18 mg for men and 13 mg for women, with an extra 2 mg during the second and third trimesters of pregnancy and an extra

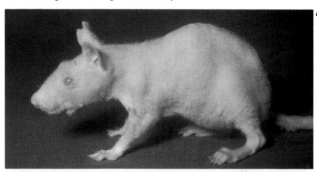
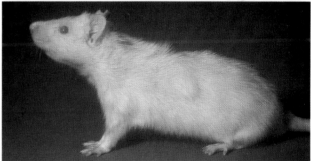
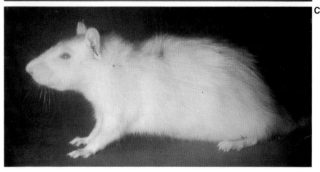

Figure 42. Skin lesions in pellagra.

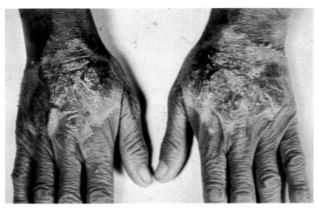

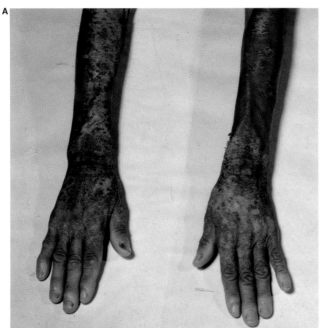

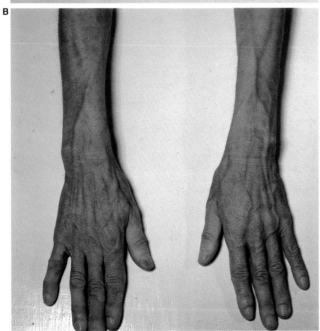

Figure 43A. Pellagrous dermatitis in advanced stage.

Figure 43B. Same patient after intensive niacin therapy.

5 mg during lactation. Children have proportionately higher requirements. An intake of 6 to 8 mg is recommended for infants, and up to 19 mg for adolescent boys.

The RDA based on caloric intake and expressed in niacin equivalents is 6.6 mg/1000 Calories and not less than 13 mg if the daily caloric intake is between 1000 and 2000.

It is believed that the minimum requirement to prevent pellagra averages 4.4 mg/1000 Calories/day, particularly if one's diet provides less than 2000 Calories.

Deficiency: A deficiency of niacin leads to the disease pellagra (Figures 42, 43, and 44).

Toxicity: Both niacin and niacinamide may be regarded as nontoxic, because there is a very wide margin between their therapeutic and toxic doses.

Niacin (but not niacinamide) acts as a vasodilator and therefore may cause flushing of the skin, dizziness, and nausea. These symptoms are temporary and in no way harmful. Because of these vasomotor symptoms, niacinamide is preferable to niacin, especially when large doses are needed for the treatment of pellagra. But, as previously mentioned, large doses of niacin lower blood cholesterol concentrations, whereas niacinamide does not have that effect.

Test of niacin status: The status of niacin, unlike that of thiamin, riboflavin, or vitamin B_6, cannot be assessed by functional tests or by tests used to measure the urinary excretion and ratio of two of its metabolites, N^1-methyl nicotinamide and N^1-methyl-2-pyridone-5-carbonylamide (2-pyridone). The classical test is simply to measure the N^1-methyl nicotinamide in urine and express it as mg/gm of creatinine. Sauberlich et al[61] gave the traditional cut-off points based on that measure.

Normally, the urine contains far more 2-pyridone than N^1-methylnicotinamide. However, with niacin restriction, the level of 2-pyridone decreases much sooner than does that of N^1-methylnicotinamide. Sauberlich et al consider ratios greater than one to be acceptable, whereas ratios below one indicate niacin deficiency.

Vitamin B_6

Vitamin B_6 is a useful term because it covers three pyridine derivatives, all of which occur in food and are interconverted metabolically in the human. These substances are pyridoxal and pyridoxamine, which are present mainly in animal products, and pyridoxine, which is present mainly in plants.

Properties: Vitamin B_6 is involved in the metabolism of amino acids and it is an essential part of the enzyme glycogen phosphorylase.

Units: The activity of pyridoxine is expressed in mg of the synthesized pure substance.

Sources: Vitamin B_6 is widely distributed in foods both of animal and of vegetable origin. Whole-grain cereals, milk, meat (especially liver and kidney), and certain vegetables are good sources of the vitamin, which is easily absorbed.

Requirements: An RDA of vitamin B_6 was first set in 1968. The allowance for adults is 2.2 mg daily plus an additional 0.6 mg daily during pregnancy and 0.5 mg during lactation.

Tests of B_6 status: The adequacy of vitamin B_6 nutriture was originally assessed by measuring the urinary excretion of tryptophan metabolites, especially xanthurenic acid, after "test loading" the patient with tryptophan.

Currently, vitamin B_6 status is assessed by measuring the degree to which added pyridoxal phosphate increases the activity of erythrocyte transaminase enzymes. As in the corresponding tests for thiamin and riboflavin, the enzyme activity is measured with and without the addition of pyridoxal phosphate. The more deficient the subject, the greater the increase in activity observed after adding the pyridoxal phosphate. The test is not yet fully standardized, but it seems that the index (activity with added pyridoxal phosphate/activity without added pyridoxal phosphate) is normally less than 1.5 for the glutamate-oxalacetate transaminase and less than 1.25 for the glutamate-pyruvate transaminase.

Deficiency: In 1949, Rinehart and Greenberg reported the experimental production of arteriosclerotic lesions in vitamin B_6 deficient monkeys, and 20 years later McCully found arteriosclerotic lesions in children dying from homocysteinuria, a rare inborn error of sulfur amino-acid metabolism. The interesting point, tying these two observations together, is that pyridoxine deficiency leads to elevated levels of homocysteine in the blood. This has led to the hypothesis that low levels of dietary pyridoxine might play a role in the genesis of atherosclerosis. In view of the contradictory results obtained by various workers, the effect of pyridoxine deficiency in atherosclerosis must at present be regarded as pure speculation.

Vitamin B_6 deficiency tends to increase oxalate excretion in the urine. Vesicle stones are prevalent in certain areas of the world where vitamin B_6 deficiency is common, eg, Thailand (Figure 45).[71] Renal calcium oxalate calculi have been treated, with some success, with magnesium oxide and vitamin B_6.

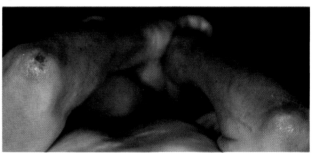

Figure 44. Nicotinamide deficiency – advanced pellagra. Dermatitis of elbows is precipitated by friction and shows initial desquamation in the center of the lesion. With periods of remission, residual pigmentation persists and becomes deeper with repeated attacks.

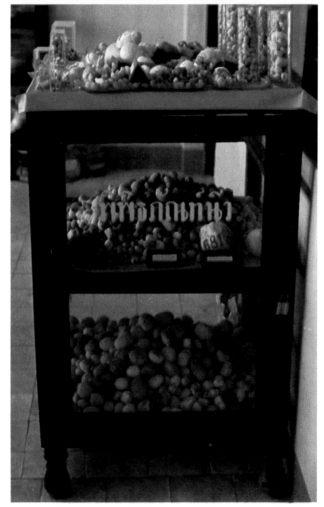

Figure 45. Oxalate bladder stones in Thailand.

Figure 46. Treatment of convulsions in pyridoxine-deficient infant.

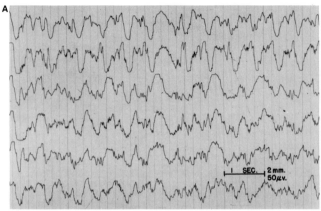

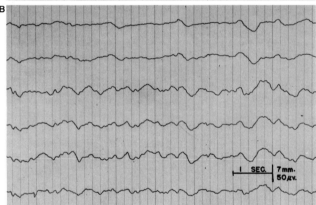

Figure 46A. Electroencephalogram of infant during convulsions produced by pyridoxine deficiency.

Figure 46B. Five minutes after pyridoxine administration; color improved and the infant slept.

Vitamin B_6 deficiency in infants is manifested by hyperirritability, convulsions, and anemia. An inborn error of metabolism leading to dependency on a high intake of vitamin B_6 has been described. It is seen during the first seven days of life and leads to convulsions (Figure 46). Unless treated early with vitamin B_6, the child may become mentally retarded. Vitamin B_6 responsive anemias have been reported to occur in adults.

Increasingly significant in clinical medicine is the vitamin B_6 deficiency that follows treatment of tuberculosis with isonicotinic acid hydrazide (isoniazid, or INH).[72] The drug leads to increased requirements for vitamin B_6, apparently by interfering with certain activities of pyridoxal phosphate. Poorly nourished patients who take isoniazid may develop severe polyneuritis, which may be both painful and disabling. Administration of pyridoxine in daily doses of 10 to 20 mg may be useful in preventing this complication of tuberculosis treatment.

There is some evidence that pregnant women develop vitamin B_6 deficiency and that supplementation may be of value in relieving the nausea of pregnancy.[73]

There is some concern about the effects of oral contraceptives on vitamin B_6 status in women. Oral contraceptives have been shown to lead to abnormalities of tryptophan metabolism, and these abnormalities can be corrected by B_6 administration.[74] It is not clear whether these metabolic changes lead to any significant clinical problems, but the matter does require further study.[75]

Experimentally induced B_6 deficiency leads to loss of appetite and weight, general weakness and lassitude, and certain symptoms and signs normally ascribed to deficiencies of other B vitamins. These include cheilosis, glossitis, peripheral neuritis, and skin changes reminiscent of pellagra.

Toxicity: Toxicity to vitamin B_6 has been reported to occur in men receiving 300 mg/day, a dose far in excess of any therapy recommended for drug treatment and a dose impossible to receive from foods.

Pantothenic Acid

Properties: Pantothenic acid is a part of coenzyme A and is a factor in the release of energy from carbohydrate. It is vital to the synthesis and degradation of sterols, fatty acids, and steroid hormones. Pantothenic acid is also involved in the acetylation of choline.

Units: The activity of pantothenic acid is expressed in mg of the synthesized pure substance.

Dietary sources: Pantothenic acid is widely distributed and is freely available in ordinary foods, so deficiency is rare in humans receiving even marginally adequate diets.

Deficiency: Hodges and others have studied volunteers on a diet deficient in pantothenic acid and including a pantothenic acid antagonist, omega methyl pantothenic acid. The subjects typically develop tiredness, abdominal pain and cramps, nausea, sometimes flatulence and vomiting, and paresthesia of the hands and feet.[76] Experimentally induced pantothenic acid deficiency in chicks results in dermatitis (Figure 47).

Malnourished World War II prisoners often developed the "burning feet" syndrome. The condition, characterized by severe paresthesia and tenderness of the feet, is believed to be in part due to pantothenic acid deficiency.

Human requirements: Probably, 4 to 7 mg of pantothenic acid daily will satisfy human requirements. Most diets in the United States, even low-cost diets, contain about 15 mg per day.

Toxicity: Toxicity to pantothenic acid is unknown in man.

Cyanocobalamin (Vitamin B₁₂)

History: The disease pernicious anemia, so named because at one time it was invariably fatal, was described in detail by Addison in England in 1849. About 50 years ago, Minot and Murphy discovered that the patient improved if he consumed raw liver. Soon after, Castle showed that beef mixed with normal gastric juice caused remission in pernicious anemia but that neither component alone was effective. Castle called the factor in the meat "extrinsic factor." He suggested that the two together interact to produce a substance, which is present in raw liver, that relieves pernicious anemia.

Not until 1948 was the anti-pernicious-anemia vitamin of liver extract finally isolated – independently, in England and in the United States. Within a very short time, cyanocobalamin (vitamin B₁₂) was shown to improve the hematological picture of pernicious anemia as well as to prevent the neurological complication of subacute degeneration of the spinal cord.

Properties: Cyanocobalamin is a red, crystalline, cobalt-containing substance that is water soluble and heat resistant. It is readily destroyed by strong acids, by alkalis, and also by sunlight. Cyanocobalamin consists of a heavy, complex, non-protein molecule. In food it is bound to protein; the intrinsic factor, an enzyme secreted by the stomach, evidently removes the cyanocobalamin from its protein combination. The vitamin is then absorbed from the small intestine and is stored in the liver and to a lesser extent in the kidney.

Figure 47A. Dermatitis in a chick whose diet was deficient in pantothenic acid. The eyelids, corners of the mouth, and adjacent skin are involved. Feathering is retarded and rough.

A

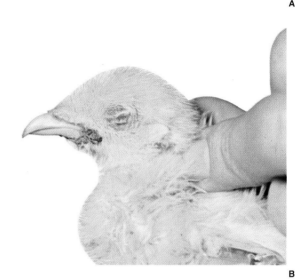

B

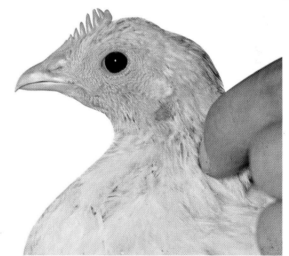

Figure 47B. Three weeks after calcium pantothenate was added to the diet, skin lesions were cured.

Cyanocobalamin is essential for the function of all cells, but particularly for cells of the bone marrow, the intestinal tract, and the central nervous system. Being active in very small amounts, it is an extremely potent catalyst that apparently facilitates reduction reactions such as the conversion of ribose to deoxyribose and of formyl through methyl reduction to tetrahydrofolic acid.[77] It also acts as a cofactor in the transfer of a methyl group to homocysteine to form methionine and in the isomerization of methylmalanyl CoA to succinyl CoA. Cyanocobalamin is probably involved in the metabolism of protein, carbohydrate, and fat, but it is of greatest importance in nucleic acid and folic acid metabolic processes.

Units: Activity of cyanocobalamin is expressed in mg and μg of the pure crystalline substance.

Dietary sources: In human diets, cyanocobalamin is obtained only from foods of animal origin, particularly meat (liver and kidney are very rich) and dairy products. It is not present in foods of vegetable origin. Herbivores obtain their cyanocobalamin from bacterial synthesis in the rumen; in human beings, however, intestinal microbial synthesis provides very little of the vitamin, because synthesis occurs in the colon, an area that does not absorb the vitamin.

Cyanocobalamin occurring in food is poorly absorbed in the absence of intrinsic factor. Storage of vitamin B_{12} in the human is good.

Human requirements: In normal adults, a diet containing 5 μg of cyanocobalamin daily will satisfy requirements. Diets in the United States show marked variation in their content of vitamin B_{12} inasmuch as the relative expense of meat, fish, and other animal products results in wide economic-class differences in the quantities consumed. High-cost diets contain about 31 μg, and low-cost diets contain as little as 2.7 μg of vitamin B_{12}. Absorption is inversely related to the intake of the vitamin, in a range from 30% to 70%.

Persons with pernicious anemia or with megaloblastic anemia due to dietary lack of cyanocobalamin often respond to as little as 0.1 μg of the vitamin given by injection.[78] Normally, 0.5 to 2.0 μg parenterally per day will maintain complete remission, but doses of 2 to 4 μg are needed to replenish liver stores. Once saturation has occurred, about 1.5 μg of cyanocobalamin daily will maintain and satisfy the biochemical needs of the body. RDAs are 5 μg for adults, 6 μg for the elderly, and 8 μg for pregnant women.

Tests of vitamin B_{12} status: Hematologically identical macrocytic megaloblastic anemias result from deficiencies of either

Figure 48. Bone marrow smears in pernicious anemia before and after vitamin B_{12} therapy.

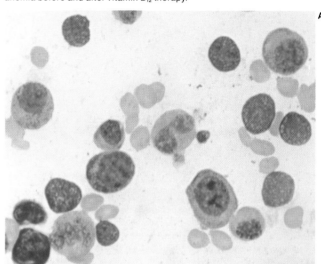

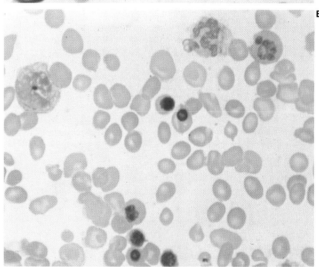

Figure 48A. Smear showing a number of megaloblasts, characteristic of certain anemias.

Figure 48B. Within 48-72 hours after treatment with 25 micrograms of vitamin B_{12} the megaloblasts have been replaced by normoblasts.

Figure 49. The tongue in pernicious anemia is typically pale and shiny, the papillae having atrophied in the course of the glossitis which is often the first symptom of the disease. The tongue may become red and sore; these symptoms usually subside promptly with therapy, but may recur in a relapse. Adequate therapy restores the tongue's normal color and may partially restore the papillae.

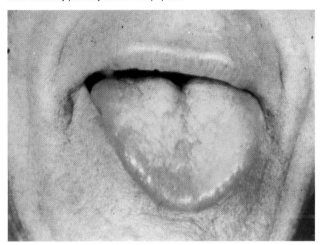

cyanocobalamin or folate; hence, one must discover which nutrient is responsible in a given patient. The ranges of erythrocyte B_{12} levels in normal subjects and in vitamin B_{12}-deficient subjects overlap, though they are lower in the deficient subjects. Therefore, the serum vitamin B_{12} level is measured, either microbiologically or using radioactive isotopes, and there is little overlap between values found in normal subjects (usually above 200 μg/ml) and those in patients with pernicious anemia (usually under 150 μg/ml).

Most patients with pernicious anemia excrete increased amounts of methylmalonic acid in urine; however, about 75% do not, even after loading with leucine or valine. Since the test is not simple to carry out, it is rarely performed as a diagnostic procedure.

Once vitamin B_{12} deficiency has been diagnosed, it is necessary to decide whether it is due to dietary deficiency or to malabsorption and, in the latter case, whether due specifically to lack of intrinsic factor or to generalized malabsorption. Malabsorption can be detected by the Schilling test, in which a small dose of radioactively labeled vitamin is given orally and then "flushed out" the next day by a large intramuscular dose of nonlabeled vitamin. A normal person will excrete at least 10% of the ingested radioactivity in his urine in the following 24 hours, whereas a person with malabsorption will excrete less, often none. If malabsorption is found, intrinsic factor is given along with radioactive vitamin, and the test is repeated. If the defect is due to lack of intrinsic factor, the test should then yield normal results.

Deficiency: Although pernicious anemia (Figure 48) is a manifestation of vitamin B_{12} deficiency, it is not due to a straightforward dietary deficiency but rather to a defect, probably genetic, that results in impaired secretion of intrinsic factor by the stomach. A consistent finding in pernicious anemia is absence or reduced amounts of both intrinsic factor and free HCl in the gastric juice. Pernicious anemia leads to weakness, to oral manifestations, and to signs of central nervous system involvement. Intermittently, the tongue becomes sore and is red and inflamed; between episodes, there is evidence of papillary atrophy (Figure 49). The tongue eventually becomes smooth and glazed. Concomitant with the glossitis are lesions of other mucous surfaces of the mouth, including the lips. The neurologic manifestations are indicative of lesions in both the lateral and posterior spinal cord, with peripheral nerve degeneration. Pallor, palpitations, and eventually more-severe cardiovascular disturbances are all features of the anemia.

76

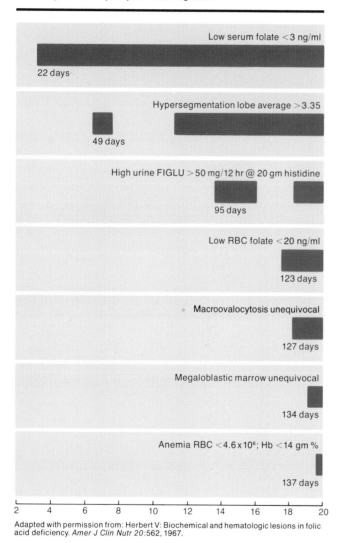

Figure 50. Hematologic and biochemical sequence of events in experimentally induced dietary folate deficiency in a healthy 35-year-old, 77 kg male.

Low serum folate <3 ng/ml

22 days

Hypersegmentation lobe average >3.35

49 days

High urine FIGLU >50 mg/12 hr @ 20 gm histidine

95 days

Low RBC folate <20 ng/ml

123 days

Macroovalocytosis unequivocal

127 days

Megaloblastic marrow unequivocal

134 days

Anemia RBC <4.6 x 10⁶; Hb <14 gm %

137 days

Adapted with permission from: Herbert V: Biochemical and hematologic lesions in folic acid deficiency. *Amer J Clin Nutr* 20:562, 1967.

Gastrectomy, if fairly radical, may cause a similar condition resulting from removal of the stomach's secreting cells.

Persons who live exclusively on vegetable products and who do not eat even dairy products and eggs are called "vegans" or "strict vegetarians." Most vegetarians, who commonly consume milk and its by-products and also eggs, are really "lacto-ovo-vegetarians." Vegans are likely to develop most of the signs of pernicious anemia, including glossitis and evidence of involvement of the long tracts of the spinal cord, but they do not necessarily develop anemia.[79] Traces of vitamin B_{12} can be ingested from fecally contaminated hands or from bacteria in soil adhering to unwashed vegetables in quantities sufficient to prevent the disorder.

Diphyllobothrium latum, the fish tapeworm, has a propensity for removing cyanocobalamin from the food in the intestine of its host. The result may be megaloblastic anemia, which can be cured by injection of the vitamin (or removal of the tapeworm).

Cyanocobalamin deficiency complicated by a deficiency of folic acid and other nutrients is a feature of sprue and other malabsorption syndromes.

Toxicity: Cyanocobalamin is not toxic to man, even when given (by mouth or injection) in amounts very much larger than those recommended for therapeutic purposes.

Folacin (folic acid, folate, and pteroylglutamic acid)
History: In the early 1930s, Dr. Lucy Wills, in India, clearly indicated the public health importance of megaloblastic anemia in pregnant women. She also demonstrated good clinical response to some antianemic principle in autolysed yeast. This principle was ineffective in addisonian pernicious anemia and was different from cyanocobalamin present in liver extract. In 1941, Mitchell and his colleagues in the United States obtained from spinach leaves a substance they called folic acid, which was important in the growth of certain microorganisms. A few years later, folic acid was synthesized and shown to have a beneficial hemopoietic effect in pernicious anemia. The immediate high hopes were diminished when it was found that folic acid did not prevent the neurological lesions of this disease.

Properties: Folic acid is a yellow substance that is slightly soluble in water. The function of folacin coenzymes is the transfer of single carbon units in intracellular synthesis, particularly of purine and serine.[80-82] Folacin is stored mainly in the liver. Blood, serum, and urine contain folacin in many different forms, and these act as growth factors for certain non-pathogenic bacteria that are normally present in the human, thus complicating physiologic studies of the vitamin.

There has been much research on the precise role of folacin in hemopoiesis. Most evidence suggests that folate deficiency anemia is extremely difficult to produce in mammals unless a folic acid antagonist is administered or certain conditions exist concurrent with the folate deficiency. These include ascorbic acid deficiency, a bacteria-free intestinal tract, or a high level of methionine added to the diet.

Units: Folacin activity is reported as mg and μg of the crystalline pure substance.

Dietary sources: Kidney, liver, vegetables, and dark green edible leaves are the richest sources of folacin in human diets. Smaller amounts are present in meat, cereals, fruits, and some roots. Milk, eggs, and poultry are poor sources. Storage of food and, particularly, cooking cause considerable vitamin loss. The vitamin is readily absorbed from the normal intestine.

Folate is found in foods in the form of polyglutamates of varying chain length. The polyglutamates must be split by "conjugase" enzymes before microbiologic analysis, and it is clear that reported values in foods are not very accurate.[83]

Human requirements: RDAs of folacin were first set by the Food and Nutrition Board in 1963. The recommendation is 0.4 mg for adults, with an additional 0.1 mg during lactation and an additional 0.4 mg during pregnancy.

Tests of folacin status: Figure 50 shows the sequence in which laboratory indices of folate deficiency occur. The hematological findings are not specific to folate deficiency inasmuch as they are identical to those of vitamin B_{12} deficiency; hence, the need for specific biochemical tests to diagnose folate deficiency.

The plasma levels of folate fall much faster than do the erythrocyte levels, but erythrocyte levels are believed to be a better index of body stores. Serum levels below 3 μg/ml are regarded as deficient; levels from 3 to 6 μg/ml, low; and levels above 6 μg/ml, acceptable. The corresponding levels for erythrocyte folate are, respectively, below 140 μg/ml, from 140 to 160 μg/ml, and above 160 μg/ml.

An interesting indirect test is based on the role of folate in the metabolism of the amino acid histidine. Histidine is broken down to formiminoglutamic acid (FIGLU) which, in the presence of adequate amounts of tetrahydrofolate, yields glutamic acid. In folate deficiency there is not enough folate to metabolize a large dose of histidine, so after oral ingestion of 15 gm of histidine, considerable amounts of FIGLU are excreted in the urine.

Deficiency: Macrocytic anemia is the main manifestation of folic acid deficiency in the human. It is characterized by alimentary tract lesions including stomatitis, glossitis, diarrhea, malabsorption, and changes in the intestines.

Megaloblastic anemia of pregnancy (Figure 51) can occur for a number of reasons: the need for folacin is increased during pregnancy, vomiting is sometimes persistent during pregnancy, the diets of some pregnant women are folacin-deficient, and, in some cases, there may be a metabolic defect in the production of the folic acid coenzymes.

In sprue and other malabsorption syndromes, there is a folate deficiency because of impaired absorption, and megaloblastic anemia is often present. Folate deficiency may also be accompanied by vitamin B_{12} deficiency.

A nutritional macrocytic anemia may occur in persons on an exceedingly poor diet (Figure 52). Megaloblastic anemia may result from deficiencies of both folic acid and vitamin C in persons with scurvy. Infants on a diet solely of milk may also develop a nutritional macrocytic anemia, because milk is deficient in both folic acid and ascorbic acid.

Megaloblastic anemia in alcoholics may be due to their generally poor dietary habits and is usually associated with low intake of folate. It has been suggested that iron deficiency may also result in a functional defect in folate utilization.

In 1962, Herbert reported on experimental self-induced folate deficiency. Four months after he had begun a low folate diet, he developed megaloblastic anemia and other signs of folacin deficiency.[84]

Perhaps no other nutrient has caused so much debate or confusion as has folacin in discussion about whether its deficiency (in man) results in disease. It is not absolutely clear whether the deficiency causes or is caused by morphological changes in the intestinal tract. The answer is probably that folacin deficiency induced by some extraneous cause is a more important public health problem than is a true dietary folacin deficiency.

Toxicity: Folacin is not toxic to the normal human even in doses much larger than those usually consumed or used therapeutically. The danger of doses greater than 0.1 mg/day is that they may mask the neurologic manifestations of pernicious anemia. Physicians who prescribe folic acid should be aware of this potential danger. In the United States it is illegal to sell without a prescription vitamin preparations that provide doses of more than 0.1 mg folic acid daily.[3]

Figure 51. Megaloblastic anemia of pregnancy treated with folic acid. Patient, 32, hospitalized with severe anemia two weeks after delivery of her fifth child, responded within 48 hours to intravenous folic acid therapy. (From the records of Boston City Hospital.)

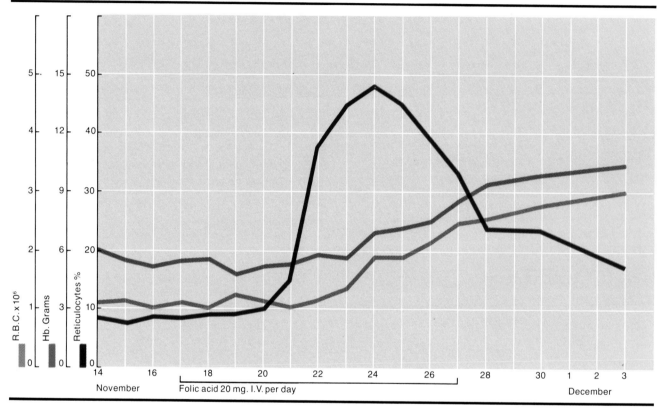

Folic acid 20 mg. I.V. per day

November   December

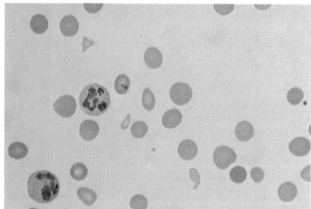

Figure 52A. Inset of peripheral blood illustrates the characteristic poikilocytosis and anisocytosis of untreated macrocytic anemia.

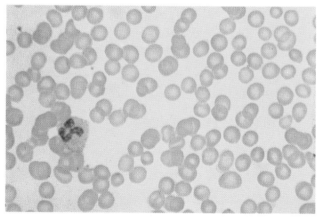

Figure 52B. Illustrates the recovery of the red cells' normal size and shape after therapy. Polymorphonuclear leukocytes, included in the photographs to indicate comparative cell size, also show, prior to treatment, the hypersegmentation typical of macrocytic anemias.

Vitamin C (Ascorbic Acid)

History: The history of vitamin C is linked with that of scurvy. Scurvy was known long before the vitamin era; the antiscorbutic effects of certain foods were described several centuries ago. In those early days, scurvy was a particular scourge of sailors who went for many weeks without fresh food. It was not until 1747, however, that James Lind of Scotland demonstrated that scurvy could be cured or prevented by the consumption of citrus fruit. Well before the discovery of vitamins, Lind's discovery led to the inclusion of certain fresh foods and fruits in sailors' diets.

In the 19th century, scurvy began to occur among infants who were being fed the newly introduced powdered and canned milks instead of the usual diet of breast milk or fresh cows' milk. The vitamin C had been destroyed when these milk products were heated during preparation.

In spite of the value attributed to vitamin C, the substance wasn't isolated until 1928 and was finally synthesized in 1932.

Properties: Ascorbic acid is a white crystalline substance very highly soluble in water and readily oxidized. It is not affected by light but is destroyed by excessive heat, especially in an alkaline solution.

Vitamin C has many functions in the body. The Food and Nutrition Board, in the 1974 *Recommended Dietary Allowances*, summarizes ascorbic acid's role in the following metabolic systems[3]:

a oxidation of phenylalanine and tyrosine via parahydroxyphenylpyruvate

b hydroxylation of aromatic compounds

c conversion of folacin to folinic acid

d regulation of the respiratory cycle in mitochondria and microsomes

e hydrolysis of alkyl monothioglycosides

f development of odontoblasts and other specialized cells including collagen and cartilage

g maintenance of the mechanical strength of blood vessels, particularly the venules

It is the failure of this latter function that leads to several of the signs and symptoms of scurvy, including hemorrhage into various tissues.

Units: Ascorbic acid is measured in mg and gm. In some textbooks it is still referred to in terms of International Units. The original IU was defined as the amount of vitamin C present in 0.1 ml of lemon juice.

Dietary sources: Vitamin C is less widely present in foodstuffs than are the other important water-soluble vitamins. In normal American diets, the main source is from citrus fruits, juices, tomatoes, and other fruits and vegetables. Eggs, meat, and fish are rather poor sources, as is milk after pasteurization. Dried cereal grains and the seeds of legumes, unless they are sprouting, are devoid of vitamin C. Vitamin C is often added to many beverages and some foods, which are so labeled.

Human requirements: The RDAs of ascorbic acid are 60 mg for adult males and females, with an additional 20 mg daily during pregnancy and an additional 60 mg daily during lactation. Recommended allowances for children range from 35 mg daily during infancy to 55 mg daily during adolescence.

These recommendations almost certainly provide a wide margin of safety; in our opinion, ascorbic acid intakes of about two thirds of the recommended allowances are more than adequate. It should be noted that in Britain the officially recommended daily allowance of vitamin C in adults is 20 mg, and in Canada, Australia, and Norway it is 30 mg. The difference of opinion is because of two schools of thought. Those favoring the higher recommendations believe in saturating the body with the vitamin, and those favoring the lesser dosage maintain that the allowance should be based on the amount required to maintain good health. There is no evidence that scurvy, poor healing of wounds, or any other abnormality occurs on intakes of 20 mg daily under conditions in which there is no increased utilization or decreased absorption of ascorbic acid.

Tests of ascorbic acid status: The most useful test of ascorbic acid status is the serum ascorbic acid level, which declines rapidly in a deficient diet. The classical cut-off points are 10 and 20 mg/dl, levels below the former being classed as deficient; between the two, low; and above 20 mg/dl, acceptable. More-recent work suggests that the levels should be raised to 20 and 30 mg/dl, respectively. Whole-blood levels are higher, and cut-offs of 30 and 50 mg/dl have been suggested.

Clinical scurvy may be related more closely to decreased ascorbate concentrations in the leukocytes than in the serum. Leukocyte ascorbate measurement may be useful in clinical settings (as opposed to population surveys). Cut-off points of 7 and 15 mg/dl have been suggested.

Figure 53. Gingival lesions in advanced scurvy.

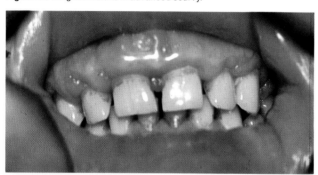

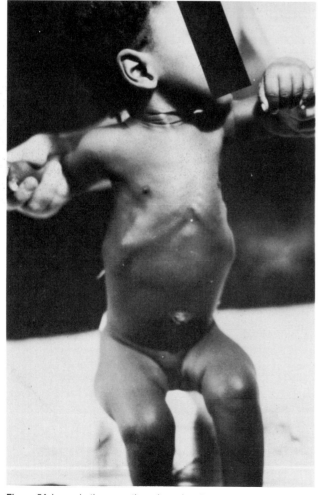

Figure 54. In scorbutic rosary, the enlarged costo-chondral junctions of scurvy resemble those of rickets. The lesions in scurvy may feel sharper and may be somewhat tender.

Deficiency: As noted on page 41, a deficiency of vitamin C leads to the disease scurvy (Figures 53 and 54). There is some evidence that a subclinical deficiency of the vitamin, not sufficient to cause any of the signs of scurvy, may result in slow healing of wounds and ulcers (Figure 55). Therefore persons undergoing surgery, those who have sustained trauma or who have persistent ulcers, and those who are suspected of having a low intake of vitamin C should have a vitamin C-rich diet or receive supplemental ascorbic acid tablets.

Claims have been made for the efficacy of large doses of ascorbic acid in preventing the common cold. Controlled trials have shown that the vitamin has no benefit in this regard.

Toxicity: Very high doses of ascorbic acid can be taken without the development of any toxic effects. After saturation is reached, the body merely excretes the vitamin in the urine. However, Herbert[85] recently suggested that very large doses ("mega doses") of ascorbic acid may destroy vitamin B_{12} in foods, and Hines[86] has suggested that some persons who take high doses of vitamin C may develop a deficiency of B_{12}.

Vitamin D

History: For many years before any knowledge of vitamin D, rickets was postulated to be a nutritional deficiency disease, and cod-liver oil had been successfully used in its treatment. It was not until 1919 that a British scientist, Sir Edward Mellanby, using puppies, demonstrated conclusively that the disease was of nutritional origin and that it responded to a vitamin present in cod-liver oil. His discovery led to some confusion, because it was already known that cod-liver oil contained vitamin A. In 1922, McCollum isolated a second fat-soluble vitamin from cod-liver oil and called it vitamin D. Around the same time, work had been proceeding that led to an explanation of how ultraviolet rays prevented rickets.

Properties: A number of compounds, all sterols, possess antirachitic properties. Certain sterols that do not possess antirachitic properties became antirachitic when exposed to ultraviolet light. The two important activated sterols are vitamin D_2 (activated ergocalciferol), which is derived from plants, and vitamin D_3 (activated cholecalciferol), which is found in animal tissues.

In human beings, when the skin is exposed to sunlight, a sterol compound (7-dehydrocholesterol) is activated to form vitamin D_3, which then becomes available to the body. This activity is identical to vitamin D ingested in the diet. The latter is absorbed from the gut only in the presence of bile.

Vitamin D promotes the absorption of calcium from the gut and is essential to the maintenance of calcium and phosphorus homeostasis and to the formation of sound teeth and bones.

Our understanding of vitamin D metabolism has been greatly increased by work done since 1969. Vitamin D is hydroxylated in the liver by an enzyme, calciferol-25-hydroxylase, to 25-hydroxy calciferol, which is further hydroxylated in the kidney to 1-25 dihydroxy calciferol, the active form of the vitamin. The synthesis of 1-25 dihydroxy calciferol is regulated by calcium levels; low levels lead to increased synthesis of the active form.[87]

Units: Vitamin D is measured in International Units. One IU is equivalent to the activity of 0.025 μg of crystalline vitamin D_2 (ergocalciferol) or 0.025 μg of pure vitamin D_3 (cholecalciferol).

Dietary sources: Vitamin D occurs naturally only in the fat of certain food products of animal origin. Eggs, cheese, milk, and butter are fairly good sources. Meat and fish contribute small quantities. Fish-liver oils are very rich in vitamin D (and vitamin A), but the amounts vary. In the United States, milk is almost uniformly fortified with vitamin D as are many other food products, especially those frequently eaten by children. The fortification of these basic foods is a very desirable public health procedure.

Human requirements: The RDA of vitamin D for children and for women who are pregnant or lactating is 10 μg (400 IU); for men and nonpregnant women, the RDA is 5 μg.

The requirement for vitamin D in adults in not really known. The amounts needed are probably so low that the requirement can be easily met by the average diet and by casual exposure to sunlight. Vitamin D requirements have been studied most extensively in infants, and it is now believed that 7 μg to 10μg (300 to 400 IU) daily permits maximum retention of calcium. Premature infants are more prone to develop rickets than are full-term infants, and their vitamin D intake should be watched. Adults, particularly aging adults, should receive an average of 400 IU daily to assist in absorption of calcium and in maintaining the calcification of their bones.

Adequate intakes of vitamin D are particularly important throughout the growth period, and the recommended allowance of 10 μg (400 IU) daily provides a comfortable margin of safety.

Any generalized statement about dietary requirements of vitamin D is difficult because of the variable contribution of vitamin D obtained from exposure of the skin to sunlight. Therefore, persons who because of their mode of life or dress

Impaired wound healing. The first satisfactory controlled experiment in human scurvy was conducted when J.H. Crandon placed himself on an ascorbic acid free diet, supplemented by all other known vitamins, for six months. After three months on the diet, when the ascorbic acid level in the blood had been zero for 44 days, a wound was made in the midback region.

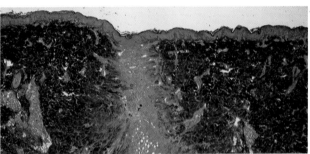

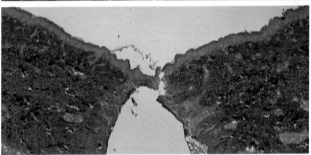

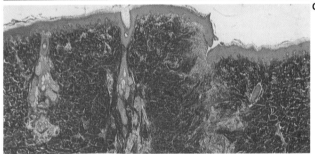

Figure 55A. Biopsy 10 days after this wound shows healing that clinically and pathologically appeared normal, but comparision with Figure 55C indicates that it was probably suboptimal.

Figure 55B. After six months of the scorbutic diet, another wound was made. Biopsy 10 days after second wound shows no healing except of the epithelium (gap in tissues was filled with a blood clot).

Figure 55C. After 10 days of ascorbic acid treatment, another biopsy of the second wound shows healing with abundant collagen formation–considerably more than occurred in the first wound.

Figure 56. Early skeletal deformities of rickets can persist throughout life. Bowlegs that curve laterally indicate that the weakened bones have bent after the second year, as the result of standing. If severe rickets occurs before the child walks, it produces a combination of bowed thighs and knock-knees.

Figure 57. The rachitic rosary is, next to cranio-tabes, the earliest sign of rickets. Enlargement of the costochondral junctions results in beads or knobs that can sometimes be seen and can always be felt or demonstrated by X-ray, as in Figure 58 (another infant).

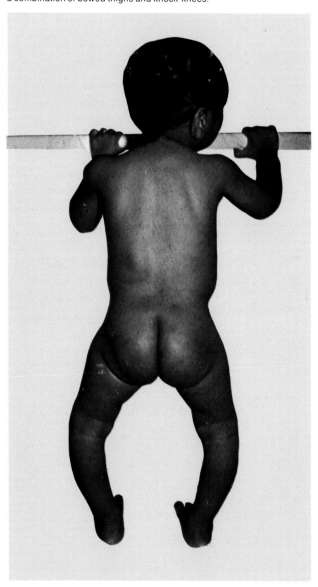

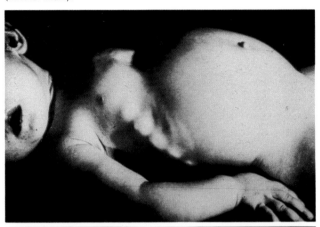

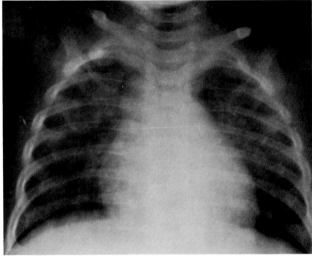

Figure 58. X-ray of infant with rachitic rosary, showing enlargement of the costochondral junctions.

receive little skin irradiation from sunlight have higher dietary needs for vitamin D. This applies to persons who work at night and sleep during the hours of sunlight, to nuns whose clothing covers most of their skin, and to persons from certain cultures such as some Muslim women who are often heavily veiled and who, along with their young children, are customarily confined indoors or in dark courtyards.

Tests for vitamin D status: Although methods for the measurement of serum 1,25-dihydroxyvitamin D_3 have been developed recently,[88] they are research procedures, not diagnostic tools. The main diagnostic tool is still the measurement of serum alkaline phosphatase concentrations which, although they are usually increased in clinical rickets, are indeterminate in the preclinical stages. Another diagnostic tool, useful in clinical practice but not in surveys, is the roentgenographic appearance of the wrist.

Deficiency: Vitamin D deficiency during childhood leads to rickets (Figures 56-58). In adults, a deficiency can result in osteomalacia.

Toxicity: Because supplementary vitamin D is added to many foods in the United States and elsewhere, intakes of vitamin D well above the RDA are common. Therefore, when vitamin D preparations are also provided medicinally, the total intake may become very high.

The fat-soluble vitamins, unlike the water-soluble vitamins, are not excreted or metabolized, and intakes greater than required tend to accumulate in the body.

Excessive quantities of vitamin D (about 2000 IU or more/kg of body weight/day) can be toxic to adults or children and may lead to hypercalcemia and its attendant complications.[89] Although some infants with hypercalcemia may be hypersensitive to vitamin D or may have an inborn error of cholesterol metabolism, many undoubtedly show a true intoxication with vitamin D. There is little rationale in exceeding the recommended daily dose of 400 IU, or 10 μg, during infancy.

In children, a common early symptom of excessive vitamin D is anorexia and vomiting. The child, though refusing food, is very thirsty and may have polyuria. Weight loss and irritability are common, and the condition may eventually lead to death. In vitamin D toxicity, the level of ionized calcium in the blood is raised. Because of the increased calcium blood level, abnormal calcification may occur in soft tissues, primarily in the walls of blood vessels but also in the kidneys, lungs, and other organs.

Vitamin E

Properties: The metabolic role of vitamin E is not fully understood, but the vitamin apparently functions as an antioxidant at the tissue level. The term vitamin E is used to mean any mixture of physiologically active tocopherols.

Dietary sources: Vitamin E is widely prevalent in foods eaten by man. The richest sources are vegetable oils. Vitamin E is also present in fresh greens and many other vegetables.

Human requirements: In the absence of definite information about human needs for vitamin E as an antioxidant, it is difficult to make a definitive recommendation of vitamin E requirements. They are believed, however, to vary between 10 and 15 mg/day for adults. The breast-fed child receives about 0.5 mg of vitamin E/kg of body weight, and this has been suggested as the minimum requirement for infants. Vitamin E requirements may be slightly increased by the consumption of polyunsaturated fats, but these fats are also good sources of the vitamin.

Deficiency: Experimentally in the rat, vitamin E deficiency often results in sterility. The female rat conceives normally but the fetuses die during gestation and are reabsorbed (Figure 59). The sterility is reversible with vitamin E therapy. In male rats, a deficiency of vitamin E leads to a permanent degeneration of testicular germinal epithelium. No similar findings have ever been described in man.

In man, the creatinuria noted in patients with cystic fibrosis and xanthomatous biliary cirrhosis has been reduced by the administration of alpha-tocopherols. A marked reticulocyte response simultaneous with a decrease in creatinuria occurred in a small series of Jordanian children suffering from protein-calorie malnutrition who were treated with vitamin E.

Experimental deficiency of vitamin E in man leads to a decrease in the levels of tocopherols in the blood, and excessive hemolysis occurs in erythrocytes that are treated with hydrogen peroxide in vitro. The clinical significance of this, if any, is not known.

The common belief among laymen that vitamin E is "the sex vitamin" and will reduce sterility and increase potency in man, or that it is useful in the prevention and treatment of heart disease, is not based on scientific fact. It is one of the falsities of nutrition information that is given wide publicity mainly by the numerous food quacks and charlatans. There is no good evidence that vitamin E has any value in lessening muscular fatigue or in the treatment of any kind of heart disease.

Reference standard: One mg of dl-alpha-tocopherol acetate

84

Resorption of fetus in a female rat with vitamin E
deficiency.

Figure 59A. Normal rat with well-developed
fetuses, 16 days pregnant.

Figure 59B. Vitamin E deficient rat at the 16th day;
uterine enlargements represent remains of autolyzed
fetuses and placentas.

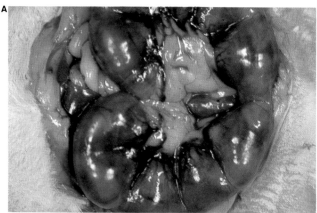

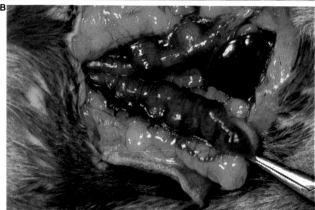

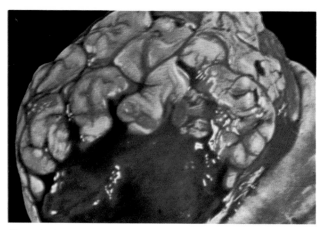

Figure 60. Hemorrhagic disease of the newborn,
resulting from vitamin K deficiency in the first few
days of life; death in this case was caused by sub-
dural hemorrhage.

is equal to one International Unit of vitamin E, according to
the National Formulary, 1965. There is no USP standard for
vitamin E.

Toxicity: Little is known about the effects of an excessive
intake of tocopherol in man, but there is some evidence of
toxicity at levels greater than 400 IU (mg)/day for prolonged
periods.

Vitamin K
Properties: Vitamin K is a fat-soluble vitamin that is necessary
for the maintenance of prothrombin, a key substance in blood
clotting. The molecular action of vitamin K remains an enigma,
but apparently it acts in the liver in the synthesis of proteins
concerned with clotting. The vitamin is believed to be active
in stimulating oxidative phosphorylation in tissues, possibly
between DPNH and a cytochrome in electron transport.

Dietary sources: Vitamin K is ubiquitous in human foods,
though in very small amounts. Most vitamin K is absorbed
after being synthesized by human bacterial flora. Dietary
deficiency in man rarely occurs.

Human requirements: The Food and Nutrition Board has not
established an RDA of vitamin K. It is believed that the small
(μg) amounts obtained from the intestinal flora and from good
food are sufficient to maintain a normal prothrombin concentration. The exception is the newborn infant who has vitamin
K deficiency in the first few days of life because its intestinal
flora is not yet well established and because the mother's
supply of the vitamin was inadequate during pregnancy.

Deficiency: Although there has been considerable debate,
it is now generally believed that vitamin K administration to
newborn infants decreases the incidence of neonatal hemorrhage, especially among premature infants or newborns with
anoxia. A single parenteral dose of 1 to 2 mg of vitamin K or one
of its analogs immediately after delivery is recommended.[90]
Infants born to mothers who are being treated with anticoagulants should receive 2 to 5 mg of vitamin K or its analog.[90]

The most serious complication of vitamin K deficiency in
infancy is cerebral hemorrhage (Figure 60). Some suggest
that the incidence could be greatly reduced by the routine
administration of vitamin K to women during the last two
months of pregnancy.

Because vitamin K is fat soluble, any defect in intestinal
absorption of fats may lead to vitamin K deficiency. Bile salts
are necessary for the absorption; an obstruction of the common bile duct may lead to a deficiency, which can result in

Egg-white injury is a deficiency produced in rats by feeding egg white, which contains a biotin antagonist, avidin.

severe bleeding following surgical intervention to relieve the obstruction. For that reason, vitamin K should be given before the operation.

In various malabsorption syndromes (sprue, celiac disease, pancreatic fibrosis, and idiopathic steatorrhea) there is poor absorption of fat and therefore of vitamin K. A similar though less severe deficiency can result from ulcerative colitis, regional ileitis, and surgical operations in which much of the intestinal tract is excised.

Toxicity: Excessive doses of synthetic vitamin K have led to hemolytic anemia and kernicterus in the infant. Newborns, therefore, should not receive doses greater than 5 mg. Moreover, 1 mg is essentially adequate so there is no reason to use such large doses.

Biotin

Biotin is essential in many enzyme systems in animals and man. The vitamin is present in many foods and is synthesized by human intestinal bacteria in sufficient quantity to satisfy normal requirements. Daily needs, probably 150 to 300 μg, are provided by most diets. Biotin deficiency does not occur in man except under very abnormal circumstances.

Raw egg white contains a substance called avidin, which, when combined with biotin, makes it unavailable to the body. Biotin prevents "egg-white injury," which is a biotin deficiency that can be produced in animals fed a diet high in egg white (Figure 61). Spontaneous biotin deficiency is an extremely rare condition that occasionally occurs in a person who, for whatever reason, has consumed a diet consisting mainly of raw eggs. It has also been reported in infants whose intestinal tract has been cleared of biotin-synthesizing bacteria by the injudicious use of sulfonamides or antibiotics. The presenting sign of biotin deficiency is an exfoliative dermatitis that responds to biotin.

Experimentally induced biotin deficiency in volunteers led to fatigue, depression, malaise, anorexia, muscle pain, nausea, signs of neuropathy, and an erythematous scaling dermatitis. These symptoms and signs disappeared when biotin was administered.

Unit standard: The activity of biotin is expressed in μg of the chemically pure substance.

Toxicity: Exceedingly large doses of biotin given to animals have not produced any toxicity. Because chemical biotin deficiency is unlikely and no therapeutic dose is recommended, biotin toxicity appears very unlikely.

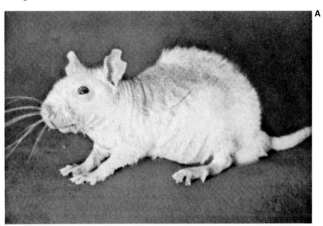

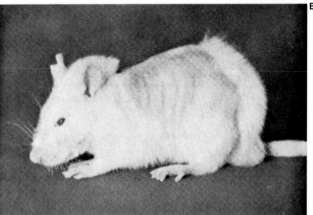

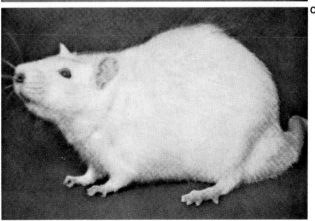

Figure 61A. The resulting dermatitis, which begins around the eyes and produces the characteristic "spectacle eye," has progressed in the rat to generalized alopecia.

Figure 61B. The same rat three weeks after adequate amounts of biotin were added to the diet. Growth has resumed and skin lesions are improved.

Figure 61C. After three months of treatment, the animal is normal.

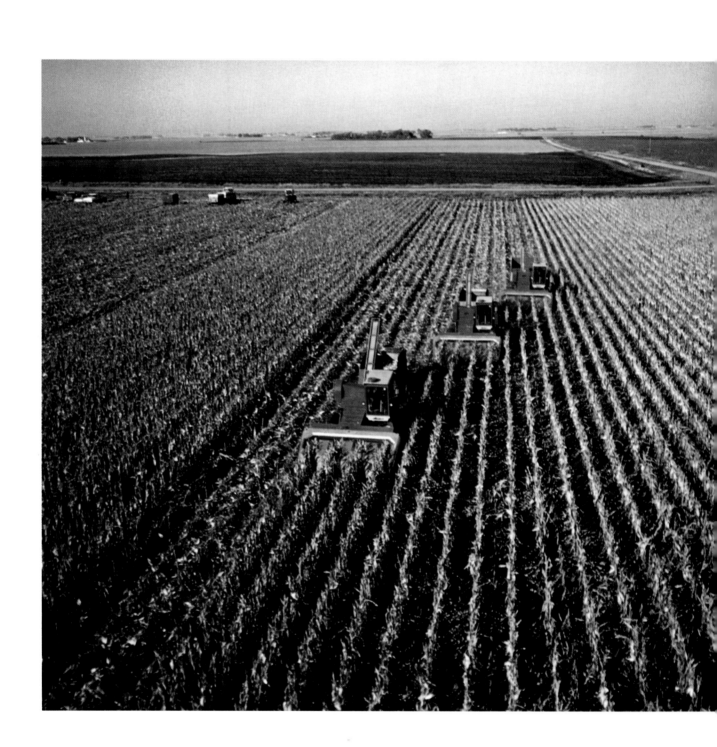

Nutritional Topics of Current Interest

NUTRITION AND INFECTION

The synergistic association between malnutrition and infectious disease has been demonstrated conclusively.[91] The consequences to the host of concurrent malnutrition and infection are more serious than those that would result from the additive effect of their independent occurrence.[92] Infections aggravate malnutrition, and poor nutritional status increases the severity of infection-caused morbidity, particularly among infants, young children, and the elderly.

Effects of Infection on Nutrition

Infection affects nutritional status in several ways. Perhaps most important is the loss of nitrogen that results from bacterial and some other infections. Nitrogen loss was first demonstrated to occur in serious infections such as typhoid fever, but has since been demonstrated in much milder infections such as otitis media, tonsillitis, chicken pox, and abscesses.

The principal mechanism by which infections cause the loss of nitrogen is probably that of increased adrenocortical activity, which mobilizes amino acids from various tissues and organs, especially muscle. The urinary excretion of nitrogen is evidence that the body is being depleted of protein.

Full recovery from an infection requires restoration of amino acids to the tissues. To achieve full recovery, therefore, the patient requires dietary intake of protein greater than normal maintenence levels. Children with diets even marginally deficient in protein, and those who are already protein-depleted, do not grow normally during and after infections. Children of poor families in many developing countries typically suffer from a quick succession of infections during the postweaning period, and often they have several infectious diseases.

Anorexia is another factor in the relation between infection and nutrition. Infections, especially if accompanied by fever or vomiting, usually cause a reduced appetite and therefore a reduced intake of food. Even when the infected patient's appetite is not impaired, he may adhere to the old adage "starve a fever." Avoiding food, or consuming only liquid, is inappropriate and may have serious consequences, especially for the child whose nutritional status is already precarious.

Intestinal parasitic infections, also, may contribute to malnutrition. Intestinal blood loss due to *Ancylostoma duodenale* and *Necator americanus* (hookworm) infections can be an important cause of iron-deficiency anemia, which is indeed prevalent where hookworm disease and iron-deficient diets are common. The fish tapeworm *Diphyllobothrium latum,* a much rarer parasite, can deprive its host of vitamin B_{12} and thereby cause megaloblastic anemia. Among the most prevalent intestinal parasites in the world, the roundworm *Ascaris lumbricoides* retards the growth of young children.

Diarrhea due to gastroenteritis is an important factor in precipitating both kwashiorkor and nutritional marasmus, and it also contributes significantly to morbidity and mortality among children in malnourished populations. Breast-fed infants are less subject to diarrhea, which is often therefore attributed to bottle-feeding or the weaning process. Actually, recent evidence suggests that many cases of childhood diarrhea may be caused by viral rather than bacterial infections. Rotaviruses (reovirus-like organisms) seem to be particularly important in that respect.[92]

Effects of Malnutrition on Infection

Considerable experimental evidence, both in man and in animals, demonstrates that dietary deficiency can reduce the body's resistance to infection. Malnourishment impairs some of the body's normal defense mechanisms. For example, children with kwashiorkor are unable to form antibodies to either typhoid vaccine or diphtheria toxoid, but the antibody-formation capability can be restored with protein therapy. Similarly, children with protein malnutrition have an impaired response to yellow-fever vaccine, and children with both kwashiorkor and nutritional marasmus have an inhibited agglutinating response to cholera antigen.

Response to the injection of vaccines is a good simulation of an organism's attack on the body, and vaccination can be done ethically (whereas experimentally induced infections with pathogenic organisms can seldom be justified in human research). Vaccination-response studies somewhat clearly indicate that the malnourished body has a reduced ability to defend itself against infection.

Leukocytosis and phagocytic activity is another defense mechanism that is impaired by malnutrition. Children with kwashiorkor show a less-than-normal leukocyte response in the presence of infection. Perhaps of great importance is the reduced phagocytic efficiency of the polymorphonuclear leukocytes in malnourished persons. The cells apparently have a defect in their intracellular bactericidal capacity. The mechanism of that defect may be related to the decreased concentrations of adenosine triphosphate observed in the leukocytes of malnourished infants, combined with decreased activity of reduced concentrations of nicotinamide adenine dinucleotide phosphate oxidase in response to phagocytic stimulation.

Although malnourished children frequently have increased concentrations of immunoglobulins (presumably related to concurrent infections), they may also have depressed cell-mediated immunity. A recent study showed the extent of that depression to be directly related to the severity of the protein-calorie malnutrition.[93] Persons with severe protein-calorie malnutrition also have low concentrations of serum transferrin that often do not return to normal for a considerable time even with proper dietary treatment.

Yet another illustration of the interaction between nutrition and infection is seen in the effect of some dietary-deficiency diseases upon tissue integrity. By reducing the integrity of certain epithelial surfaces, notably the skin and mucosa, malnutrition decreases the host's resistance to invasion by pathogenic organisms.

BREAST-FEEDING AND BOTTLE-FEEDING OF INFANTS
Most infants in the United States and other western industrial countries are bottle-fed rather than breast-fed, although there is a trend toward nursing. Increasing numbers, though still a minority, of American infants are now breast-fed for at least three to four months. In many poor, developing countries, mothers generally still nurse their infants, often beyond the time of infancy (one or two years). The increasing practice of bottle-feeding in those countries, however, may create grave health problems for children of poor families.

The food industry has developed infant-feeding formulas or breast-milk substitutes, most of which are based on cow's milk, that are nutritionally quite similar to human milk. Although manufacturers claim to have "humanized" those products by the addition of all nutrients necessary for human growth, human milk is still unique in that it contains immunoglobulins and other components that may confer immunity or protect the infant against infection.[94] Both colostrum and breast milk provide a number of anti-infective factors such as immunoglobulins, various cells (macrophages and lymphocytes), and supernatant substances (including antibody, complement, lysozymes, lactoferrin, and interferon).

For economically secure mothers and their infants who live in sanitary environments, bottle-feeding generally poses no great danger to health, but neither does it provide any therapeutic advantages. Mothers everywhere should be encouraged to breast-feed rather than to bottle-feed their babies for at least six months, unless they have some good reason for not doing so and can be expected to safely bottle-feed. The advantages of nursing include its convenience, the adequacy of nutrients in breast milk, a reduced likelihood of obesity in the infant, the low cost, the good mother-child relationship that nursing fosters, the immunity to disease conferred by the constituents of breast milk, and the fact that the infant's susceptibility to diarrhea is decreased by breast-feeding (and increased by bottle-feeding).

A further consideration, especially in nonindustrial cultures, is that full lactation delays the return of ovulation,[95] often for eight months or more. The infant's sucking stimulus maintains high maternal serum prolactin concentrations, which in turn suppress ovarian function and gonadotropin release. Breast-feeding is clearly not a reliable method of birth control, but even when no other contraceptive methods are practiced, intervals between pregnancy are about six to nine months longer among lactating mothers than among nonlactating mothers. In some countries, fertility rates are being affected more by breast-feeding than by all artificial birth-control methods combined. The increasing practice of bottle-feeding in those countries can therefore be expected to intensify the problem of overpopulation by leading to closer spacing of children.

In the United States and other industrial countries, some concern has been expressed that toxic substances (such as DDT or PCB) consumed by the mother may be secreted in her milk. DDT was once the main concern, but now there is more concern about PCB. There is little current evidence to suggest that dangerously high levels of PCB are present in the milk of women not specifically exposed to them for long periods of time. It must be remembered that cow's milk and other foods may be contaminated as well, and there is little evidence that the milk of mothers not especially exposed to those chemicals contains dangerously high concentrations over long periods of time. The long-term answer to the problem is of course environmental protection – not the abandonment of breast-feeding. Physicians and the public must rely on regulatory agencies to monitor the problem and to provide information and guidance in particular situations.

Problems for Poor Families in Developing Countries

For poor families in developing countries especially, the two primary health problems related to bottle-feeding are (a) nutritional marasmus or other forms of severe malnutrition and (b) gastroenteritis.[95] Both conditions contribute to high rates of infant mortality in "third-world" countries.

Typically, for economic reasons or because the mother cannot read instructions, the relatively expensive powdered milk or formula is overdiluted. The overdiluted formula does not supply enough nutrients or calories to permit normal growth, and, if the infant receives no other food, he may develop nutritional marasmus or other signs of malnutrition.

The pediatric wards of hospitals in tropical countries are full of babies dying from gastoenteritis, which is extremely common among bottle-fed infants wherever proper hygiene is difficult or impossible to maintain. Milk is a good vehicle and culture medium for pathogenic organisms. When it is reconstituted with water from a contaminated ditch or well and cannot be stored in a refrigerator, it might be considered liquid pestilence. A clean formula (much less a sterile one) is incredibly difficult to provide when the family water supply is a contaminated ditch or well, when household hygiene is poor and the family lives among flies and dung, when there is no refrigerator or other safe storage place for mixed formula, where fuel must be gathered to boil water, and when the uneducated mother has very little understanding of the "germ" concept of disease.

The Decline in Breast-Feeding

The practice of bottle-feeding in poor communities of nonindustrial countries is increasing for a number of reasons. In some areas, bottle-feeding has become a status symbol: that is how babies are fed in wealthy societies; the influence of western culture is seen in the portrayal of breasts as sex objects rather than functional anatomic organs; and bottle-feeding formulas have been advertised and promoted aggressively.

Moreover, the medical profession itself has not generally recognized the advantages of breast-feeding[96]; some medical students are still inadequately instructed in proper infant nutrition. Hospitals and medical training in developing countries tend to follow the practices of western industrial countries, and in many hospitals throughout the world, babies are bottle-fed and mothers are even discouraged form nursing. Some physicians and nurses help to create concern in mothers about their ability to successfully breast-feed their infants.

Although psychological factors can undoubtedly influence the "let-down" reflex and the mother's supply of milk, lactation failures are strikingly few in traditional societies where nursing is the normal practice and is publicly acceptable.

Mothers in the United States and certain other countries can get useful information and peer support for breast-feeding from local branches of LaLeche League,* an organization that provides medically sound information on the subject. Their publications are useful not only to mothers but to the medical profession as well.

NUTRITION IN THE HOSPITAL

During the past decade, physicians have become increasingly aware that varying degrees of malnutrition, particularly protein-calorie malnutrition, may be relatively common among patients in hospitals.[97] Many patients have a significant degree of malnutrition secondary to other diseases such as neoplasms, and most patients, even those who are admitted in an optimal nutritive state for an elective procedure, are subjected to various stimuli, treatments, conditions, and stresses that affect the body's homeostasis and, therefore, nutritional requirements. Stress, no matter what its cause — emotional, traumatic, or physiologic — stimulates a series of neuroendocrinologic and metabolic changes that alter the metabolism of protein, carbohydrate, fluid, and electrolytes. Furthermore, stress is often accompanied by anorexia.

The reason for concern about "hospital malnutrition" is the increasing evidence that it has a great impact upon morbidity and mortality. Nutritional therapy may therefore be a primary component contributing to the effectiveness of many medical and surgical procedures. That fact has been dramatized by the advent of successful total parenteral nutrition. Positive nitrogen balance, spontaneous closure of fistulas, weight gain, and more-rapid healing of surgical wounds are among the results of total parenteral nutrition.

The interest in "hospital malnutrition" has led to the establishment of multidisciplinary nutrition committees in many hospitals. The committees, which typically include physicians, dietitians, nutritionists, pharmacists, and physical therapists, promote optimal nutrition for all hospital patients. They also provide consultation services and supervise nutritional therapy for selected patients.

Nutrition affects many components of the body's complex defense system against infection. For example, malnutrition can compromise the integrity of the skin and mucous mem-

*LaLeche League International, Franklin Park, Illinois 60131.

branes, the natural barriers that normally risk penetration by microorganisms. Malnutrition can also impair defenses such as immunoglobulin-A (IgA), phagocytosis, and cell-mediated immunity (CMI). Nutritional therapy in adults can often revert depressed CMI reactions to normal. The impact of infection on the patient's nutritional status should be considered, and nutritional support should be included as part of the patient's treatment plan.

Even relatively mild and self-limited infections produce a host of metabolic changes, including hypermetabolism and ·increased loss of nutrients. The combination of hypermetabolism and anorexia can produce weight loss. Body defense mechanisms mobilized in response to invasive microorganisms further increase nutritional needs. For example, protein requirements are increased to meet the demands for antibody synthesis and for the formation of phagocytic and lymphoid cells. To replenish the catabolic losses that accompany even brief febrile periods may require dietary supplementation for several weeks after body temperature and laboratory test results have returned to normal. Two laboratory tests that are useful as indicators of both protein-calorie malnutrition and CMI status are the measurements of serum albumin and transferrin concentrations. Skin tests with recall antigens (*Candida*, streptokinase/streptodornase, mumps) are also commonly used to evaluate CMI.

Because hospital malnutrition is common, physicians should have the expertise to assess nutritional status and to recommend nutritional therapy as needed. A complete nutritional assessment includes clinical, biochemical, and dietary components. The findings in one component, eg, laboratory-test results, should be interpreted in conjunction with those in the other components of assessment.

The method most commonly used to assess dietary intake is a 24-hour diet recall plus a history of the frequency of intake of certain foods. Further useful information for nutritional counseling includes the patient's food likes and dislikes, weight history, and use of special diets, medications, and vitamin or mineral supplements.[98]

FOOD FADDISM

Faddism, quackery, and charlatanism in food and nutrition have been around a long time and no doubt will continue to be. Basically this is because everyone thinks he is an authority on food because all of us eat. We all have had various personal experiences (both good and bad) with food and we want to share these experiences with others. Some want to share them for a fee and with a little exaggeration. But this is not scientific nutrition; it is testimonial, hearsay, fantasy, and (for a few) a lucrative business.

Dictionaries define a fad as a silly thing followed with an exaggerated zeal. A quack is a pretender to skill, particularly in health and medicine, and a charlatan is a quack who is also a vendor of remedies.

Faddism, quackery, and charlatanism exist all over the world, from primitive huts in the jungle to plush suites on Park Avenue. They are characterized by countless numbers of bizarre diets to lose weight, by the use of many-colored pills for reducing (some combinations of which are truly dangerous), by tonics, and by nutritional supplements claimed to increase appetite and "build one up." Food faddism is particularly rife among trainers and athletic coaches, from high school through professional teams.

Vitamin C, vitamin E, and food referred to as natural, organic, health, macrobiotic, and Dr. So and So's quick-weight-loss diets are all vying for top place on the totem pole of nutritional nonsense. We all need vitamin C – 30 to 45 mg daily – and we easily get that amount from a diet that includes a little citrus fruit or tomatoes. But doses of 500, 1000, or 10,000 mg daily are pure quackery. These huge amounts will not decrease one's susceptibility to the common cold or any other disorder, and they may carry potential harm. We all need vitamin E in amounts varying from 10 to 25 IU daily, and we easily get that amount from a varied diet. Amounts of 100, 500, or 1000 IU per day will not prevent or treat any kind of heart disease, sexual impotence, muscle cramps, or anything else.

So-called natural, organic, and health foods currently are having quite a rebirth in food quackery. All foods are natural or made from natural foods, but this is not the same as saying that all nutrients are natural. For example, vitamin C is natural as it is found in citrus fruits and is synthetic when added to many noncitrus juices or drinks, but in both cases it is identical in chemical composition and physiologic action. To paraphrase Gertrude Stein, "vitamin C is vitamin C is vitamin C." So-called imitation meats are usually made from textured soybean protein and hence are also made of a natural food.

All foods are "organic" in that they are made of organic compounds: carbon, hydrogen, and oxygen. All foods are "health foods" in that as part of a balanced diet they contribute to health.

But what the devotee (or promoter) of natural, organic, or health foods has in mind are foods grown with the aid of manures and composts rather than chemical fertilizers; foods grown without the use of chemical pesticides; and foods not processed with the aid of chemical additives such as preservatives, antioxidants, and various flavoring and coloring agents. Some people believe that such foods are more healthful, but there is not a shred of evidence to support their beliefs or the testimonials they are so eager to give. There is increasing concern that much food quackery is filled with chicanery and fraud because of the high profits to be reaped.

Macrobiotic means "large or long life" but the original macrobiotic diets ("Zen macrobiotic diets"), based largely on brown rice and severe restriction of fluid, cause just the opposite. The medical literature contains documented evidence of severe ill health and even death caused by following such nutritional nonsense to the extreme. Macrobiotic diets are usually combined with a certain amount of pseudo-oriental philosophy that seems to give the diets an aura they do not deserve. Modern "macrobiotic diets" do not restrict fluid and are not limited to very few foods. They are essentially lacto-ovarian vegetarian diets and are compatible with good health.

Whereas macrobiotic diets have taken their place in food faddism only in recent times, the so-called Mayo Diet has been around for more than a generation. Let us emphasize that this diet is usually referred to as the Mayo Diet, not the Mayo Clinic Diet. It did not originate with the Mayo Clinic and has been a constant source of embarrassment to that well-respected institution.

What is the Mayo Diet? "Eggs, bacon, and grapefruit, all you can eat, but nothing else, and we guarantee you will lose weight. The grapefruit has peculiar and special properties that help burn up fat, including stored body fat, so that calories are lost." What nutritional nonsense! Grapefruit is a good citrus fruit but it is no big yellow spark plug that metabolizes fat. We think the Mayo Diet is dangerous because eggs and bacon contain a large amount of saturated fat and cholesterol.

The many "quick-weight-loss diets," even though some are promoted by physicians, have no scientific validity. True, one will lose weight because of the sheer boredom of eating the very limited choice of foods or because of the nauseating effect of the usually high fat content of the diets. But quick-weight-loss diets do not train one in proper eating habits. They offer

too much saturated fat. They do not provide good nutrition. They do not stress the equally important need for more physical activity (exercise) in achieving weight loss. Weight is promptly regained when one goes off these "odd-ball" diets. They are another example of contemporary quackery and charlatanism. Recent entries in the "fad parade" are the liquid protein diets; the liquid hydrolyzed protein diets are downright dangerous.

One must learn to live *with* food, not *without* it!

Three relatively recent books effectively deal well with food faddism: *The New Nuts Among the Berries* by Ronald M. Deutsch (Bull Publishing Company, Palo Alto, 1977) is a "classic" on food faddism. *The Health Robbers*, edited by Stephen Barrett, MD, and Gilda Knight, with a foreword by Ann Landers (Philadelphia, Stickley, 1976), deals not only with food faddism but also with many other types of health quackery. *Panic in the Pantry – Food Facts, Fads, and Fallacies*, by E. M. Whelan and F. J. Stare (New York, Atheneum, 1977), is a popular, humorous, and easily read book.

LACTOSE INTOLERANCE
Lactose, a disaccharide, is the sugar in milk, and lactase is the intestinal enzyme necessary for its metabolism. If the quantity of lactase is low (or absent), lactose cannot be metabolized and thus absorbed. It slowly passes through the bowel, where the normal bacterial flora ferment it to organic acids, thus changing the pH of the stool. Gas is formed, an osmolar flow of water is directed into the intestine, and the lactase-deficient patient has considerable abdominal distress often accompanied by diarrhea.

An intolerance to lactose should not be confused with gastrointestinal milk allergy. This latter condition results from a sensitivity to milk, usually to the milk protein beta-lactoglobulin. The disease manifests itself in early infancy and the prevalence is low, probably less than 1%.

In contrast, lactose intolerance is more prevalent and is seen mainly in older children or even adults. In nearly all humans, lactase activity is high in infancy. However, in the nonwhite races, as in most other mammals, lactase activity often drops to low levels after weaning and remains low throughout adulthood. Most whites (and possibly persons of some other races) who continue to drink milk beyond infancy have high levels of the enzyme throughout life.

Lactase deficiency, which is more correctly termed low-lactase activity, is of three types:

1. *Congenital lactase deficiency.* This is a rare clinical condition in which diarrhea develops soon after birth.[99] The failure to utilize lactose leads to malnutrition and wasting. If diarrhea persists and is accompanied by vomiting, there is a loss of fluid and electrolytes. When the milk is withdrawn and replaced by a lactose-free diet, the diarrhea disappears and the infant begins to thrive.

2. *Secondary low-lactase activity.* A reduced level of intestinal lactase activity is often found secondary to other disease states in which there is damage to the microvilli of the brush border of the intestinal mucosa.[100] Many gastrointestinal diseases affect intestinal enzyme activity in this manner. In developing countries, diarrheal disease and protein-calorie malnutrition are important causes of reduced disaccharidase activity.

3. *Primary low-lactase activity.* This is a relatively common condition in nonwhite populations in the United States and other parts of the world.[101] In people with this condition, milk was usually well tolerated in early childhood (presumably because of high levels of lactase activity), but in later childhood and in adulthood, levels of the enzyme are low. The condition cannot be termed an abnormality or disease, because it is found in 80% to 90% of persons of Asian or African origin, in most other nonwhite peoples, in 5% to 20% of whites, and in practically all mammals, including the nonhuman primates.

Lactase activity is usually assessed either by a lactose-load test followed by serial measurements of any rise in blood glucose above the fasting level or by intestinal biopsy and determination of enzyme activity levels in the mucosal specimen.

Symptoms and signs are similar whether the lactose intolerance is congenital, primary, or secondary. They include abdominal pain or cramps, diarrhea, and flatulence or bloating. These signs frequently occur in persons with low levels of enzyme activity soon after consumption of 50 gm of lactose, the amount usually given in the fasting state in adult lactose-load tests. Some of these subjects may also have similar symptoms when they drink milk.

Evidence suggests that many persons with low lactase activity can consume milk without any problems arising.[102] A recent study showed that all the adult subjects investigated who had flat lactose curves could consume at least one cup of milk and most could consume far more at one sitting without developing undue symptoms.[103] This freedom from symptoms may be due to the development, over time, of a tolerance to unabsorbed lactose and the products of its breakdown in the intestinal tract. Whatever the mechanism, it seems that milk is not contraindicated as a useful dietary supplement even in populations where low levels of lactase activity are prevalent. It is advisable, however, to be aware that symptoms of intolerance could arise and to introduce milk in gradually increasing amounts.

THE ROLE OF FIBER IN THE DIET

Recently it has been claimed, even by some physicians, that a lack of fiber in the American diet is in part responsible for several common diseases. These include diverticular disease, cancer of the colon, appendicitis, irritable bowel syndrome, coronary heart disease, hemorrhoids, varicose veins, and others. Most of the scientific comments on this subject have emanated from England, from the writings of Burkitt, Trowell, Painter, and Cummins et al. Many of their conclusions are based on associations between disease prevalence and diets of population groups, and in only a few instances on controlled experiments. As to be expected, charlatans have jumped into the fiber fury with exaggerated claims and popular books for the gullible.

Fiber is defined as that part of plant material in our food that is resistant to digestion. Fiber includes carbohydrate compounds such as cellulose and hemicelluloses, and a noncarbohydrate substance, lignin.

A high-fiber diet increases fecal bulk, produces more-frequent bowel movements with softer stools, and decreases transit time through the intestine. Presumably, the increased bulk due to fiber mechanically stimulates the intestinal tract. A high-fiber diet can therefore be used safely to treat constipation and has none of the adverse side effects of most laxatives.

During the past hundred years in the western hemisphere, there has been a decrease both in the fiber content of flour used for baking and in the amount of bread consumed. This is due in part to milling and to an increased consumption of fats, sugar, and animal products. During the same period there has been a marked increase in diverticular disease, which was rare before 1920 and is now a common colonic disorder in North America and Europe. In countries where the fiber content of the diet has remained high, however, diverticular disease is rare.

Burkitt[104] believes that the difference in prevalence of diverticular disease is because persons on refined diets pass stools that are small, hard, and have a long intestinal transit time. In contrast, persons on a high-fiber diet have more bulky, soft stools, which pass through the intestine more rapidly. The refined diet results in relatively long periods of contact between the mucosa and the intestinal contents, and in strained defecation. The straining is believed to lead to hypertrophy of the bowel muscle, a tendency to pouching, and a greater likelihood of irritation and inflammation once diverticuli have formed.

In a study by Painter et al, 70 patients with diverticular disease of the colon were treated with a high-fiber diet including unprocessed bran.[105] Follow-up for an average of 22 months showed relief of symptoms in 62 patients. However, there was no control group, and the only established criteria of therapeutic effect depended on patients' descriptions of their own symptoms. Before this method of therapy can be generally recommended for treatment of diverticular disease, a controlled trial using quantitative methods is needed.

Arteriosclerosis and coronary heart disease may also be related to a low-fiber intake. Trowell suggests that a high-fiber intake lowers blood cholesterol concentrations by increasing fecal steroid output, which is the main catabolic pathway for cholesterol in man.[106] An association is found between populations whose mean serum cholesterol levels are low, who have relatively little atheromatous disease, and whose diet is customarily high in fiber. Animal studies in part support this evidence. But, as has been discussed earlier in this book, other dietary and nondietary factors have important positive associations with raised serum cholesterol levels and a high incidence of coronary heart disease. These risk factors include diets high in total calories, saturated fats, and cholesterol; lack of exercise; obesity; hypertension; diabetes; cigarette smoking; and a family history of early-onset coronary heart disease.

Low intakes of dietary fiber have been linked with colonic cancer, appendicitis, and the irritable bowel syndrome.[107] Again, the evidence is based mainly on inconclusive epidemiological data showing a low incidence of these diseases in Africa as compared with Europe and North America, and changes over time in the latter continents. Varicose veins, hemorrhoids, and venous thrombosis in the legs may be produced by pressure on veins returning from the affected areas. Chronic constipation or frequent strained defecations may play a role in the etiology of these conditions.

Foods that contain fiber include whole grains, lightly milled wheat, rice and corn products, bran-containing breakfast cereals, and most fresh fruits and vegetables. By increasing the consumption of those foods, it is easy to increase appreciably the fiber content of the diet. However, the beneficial effects of a high-fiber diet in preventing disease needs further research and documentation.

DRUG-AND-NUTRIENT INTERACTIONS[108, 109]

Drugs can affect nutritional status in any of three ways, by influencing (a) appetite, (b) absorption, and (c) metabolism.

The best known drug that increases the appetite is alcohol, taken in moderation before a meal. Insulin and the sulfonylureas also increase appetite, as perhaps do sex hormones. The appetite of depressed patients is improved by antidepressants, and that of hypothyroid patients by thyroid medication. None of these drugs are used primarily for their effects on appetite.

Drugs that reduce appetite are either designed for the purpose (anorectic drugs) or do so as an undesirable side effect. The former group includes bulk agents and amphetamines and compounds related to the amphetamines. The latter group includes bad-tasting drugs such as chloral hydrate, paraldehyde, some vitamin B preparations, and others excreted in saliva into the mouth, such as potassium iodide and bromide-containing medications. None of these drugs are very useful in reducing appetite, and amphetamines can be hazardous and are frequently contraindicated.

Many drugs cause steatorrhea and malabsorption of several nutrients. The intestinal mucosa appears to be harmed by some drugs such as neomycin, kanamycin, colchicine, and para-amino salicylic acid. Cholestyramine will bind bile salts and hence lead to decreased absorption of fats, and liquid paraffin (mineral oil) can interfere with the absorption of fat-soluble vitamins. Beta-sitosterol will decrease cholesterol absorption, an obviously desirable effect. Other drugs that affect absorption are discussed by Hartshorn.[108]

A large number of drugs can affect nutrient metabolism. Diuretics, adrenal corticosteroids, and purgatives can lead to potassium depletion; corticosteroids, oral contraceptives, and other drugs can lead to sodium retention; and sulfonylureas and phenylbutazone can decrease iodide uptake by the thyroid.

Many vitamins can be affected by drugs. Thiamin deficiency in chronic alcoholism, riboflavin deficiency induced by isoniazid, and megaloblastic anemia accompanying anti-convulsant therapy have been known for a long time. Another well-documented effect is that of prolonged antibiotic administration on vitamin K, leading to an undesirable depression of prothrombin levels and the therapeutic depression of prothrombin levels by anticoagulants.[108]

Monoamine oxidase (MAO) inhibitors, used as antidepressants, interact indirectly with foods rich in tyramine, a substance that can lead to the release of norepinephrine from intraneuronal storage sites. Normally, it is destroyed by MAO in the small intestine, but in MAO-inhibitor-treated patients it may be absorbed, leading to severe autonomic reactions. The most important source of tyramine is "old" cheese, but it is widely distributed (in lower concentrations) in other foods.

A different effect of drugs on nutrition is that certain drugs contain a fair amount of sodium. This is of special importance in patients on low-sodium diets.

Much interesting work is being done on the effects of the nutritional state on drug metabolism. Many drugs are detoxified by the microsomal mixed-function oxidases, whose activity is depressed by prolonged protein malnutrition. In animals, a fat-free diet will also depress the activity of these enzymes. Chronic alcohol ingestion, on the other hand, will stimulate the microsomal oxidases. It is not clear what the clinical significance, if any, of these findings is.

A final consideration is that some foods can affect the absorption or efficacy (bioavailability) of certain drugs. The subject is of increasing interest to pharmacologists and should be considered in prescribing drugs and diets.

DIETARY GOALS FOR THE UNITED STATES

The Senate Select Committee on Nutrition, known as the McGovern Committee, was terminated December 31, 1977, and became a part of the larger Committee on Agriculture. In February 1977, it issued a report entitled *Dietary Goals for the United States*.[110] The report recommended six goals:

1 Increase carbohydrate consumption to account for 55% to 60% of the energy (caloric) intake.

2 Reduce overall fat consumption from approximately 40% to 30% of energy intake.

3 Reduce saturated fat consumption to account for about 10% of total energy intake, and balance that with polyunsaturated and monounsaturated fats, which should account for about 10% of energy intake each.

4 Reduce cholesterol consumption to about 300 mg/day.

5 Reduce sugar consumption by about 40% to account for 15% of total energy intake.

6 Reduce salt consumption by about 50% to 85% to approximately 3 gm/day.

The Goals have been criticized by many physicians and nutritionists[111,112] who complain that, in general, the Committee report frequently states as established fact observations that can be described, at best, as rumor and speculation. The report, they claim, frequently overlooks reality, namely that eating is more than a biologic experience and is indeed a pleasure of life.

The Goals were slightly revised early in 1978[113] and fortunately gave more emphasis to the hazards of obesity and the increasing role of alcohol in providing calories in American diets. Although the basic criticism of the Dietary Goals still stands, the Goals have brought nutrition to the attention of the Congress and the public; that, indeed, is important.

At the time of this writing, the Goals are being further revised by representatives from the Departments of Agriculture and Health, Education, and Welfare. Because the version is being prepared by well-qualified nutritionists rather than nonprofessional Senate staff members, it will be a far sounder document. An important step in that direction was the publication, in December 1979, of the American Society for Clinical Nutrition on the evidence relating to the Goals.[114]

NUTRITION IN A WORLD WITHOUT PLENTY

The world is short of food, and the shortage is increasing. Largely this is because there are more mouths to feed every year, and there will be for many more years. Thus, it makes good sense not only to redouble our efforts for population control but also to increase the production and dietary use of the most efficient and least expensive source of calories. That is not because one can live or even exist from calories alone, but rather because one cannot live, be productive, or be happy without sufficient calories; with adequate calories, protein is spared, work can be done, and life can be more pleasant.

We must depend on agriculture to produce food, but the chemist can improve many of our basic foods by means of appropriate fortification. For example, the essential amino acid lysine can be added to wheat products in countries where other foods do not provide adequate lysine, and the essential amino acids lysine and threonine can be added to rice in countries where other foods do not provide them in adequate amounts. Similarly, water can be fortified with fluoride, margarine and low-fat milks with vitamins A and D, noncitrus juices with vitamin C, refined white flour with some of the B vitamins and iron, and salt with iodide. A recent example is the fortification of sugar with vitamin A in various parts of the world.

The chemist can nutritionally improve certain basic foods at far less cost than the farmer can provide other appropriate foods to lessen nutritional deficiencies; most important, with fortification, food habits do not have to be changed, a very difficult and time-consuming task.

We need more food – both in the developed and the developing countries. Intensive efforts are necessary both for increasing the crop yield in each agricultural acre and for reducing food deterioration and waste. Additionally, however, it is apparent that we need new sources of food; attention is being given to synthesizing new sources of nutrients, and there is optimism about scientific progress in the area of fortifying the biological value of certain plant proteins. One should remember that the farmer and the chemist together can do a better job of solving the problems of global nutrition than either can do alone.

The world is short of food because of our failure to effectively slow the rate of population increase, and because of our waste. We must and will consume fewer animal foods and more cereals, potatoes, and sugar – the latter being only calories but yet the most-efficient and least-expensive source of calories. We need increased research in agriculture and food technology and we need public understanding and legislation to encourage such research. Food is not only necessary to survive; it is among the pleasures of life.

To achieve a world with plenty of food, we need enlightened, realistic, and common sense views in our governmental regulatory and environmental agencies. The proper use of pesticides and insecticides on crops, antibiotics in animal feeds, and food additives to prevent spoilage of foods is vital to producing enough food. The potential risks of using these substances must be carefully weighed against the benefits – indeed their necessity. So far the benefits have, in our opinion, far outweighed the risks. These situations must be carefully and continuously monitored by industry and our regulatory agencies, but too often the emotions of noisy activists and a few publicity-seeking scientists are more persuasive with governmental agencies than are scientific facts.

Finale

Now that many of our more serious infectious diseases can be prevented, controlled, and well treated, good nutrition is recognized as a most important factor influencing our health and indeed as an important part of treating certain diseases.

Cardiovascular disease is today the most-frequent cause of death, and nutrition is importantly concerned with the prevention and treatment of both atherosclerosis and hypertension, two of the most common diseases in this category. Certain types of cancer are associated with nutritional habits, generally "overnutrition" and high-fat diets. The use of fluoride to prevent dental caries has been one of the great nutritional and public health triumphs of recent years, yet much remains to be done educationally to make this discovery as effective as it should be. Many children still do not receive adequate amounts of fluoride, and iron-deficiency anemia, one of the first deficiency diseases to be recognized, is still common in the United States.

In other parts of the world, primarily the underdeveloped areas, major health problems directly concerned with improper or poor nutrition include lack of total calories, protein-calorie malnutrition of early childhood, a host of infectious diseases made worse by poor nutrition, iodide-deficient goiter, anemias due not only to a lack of iron but also to lack of folic acid, and blindness due to lack of vitamin A.

It does seem strange that instruction in nutrition was so slow to get started in most of our medical, dental, public health, and nursing schools. Why? Perhaps because historically, and even until recently, emphasis has been on getting sick people well, not keeping well people well. (For example, the President's Commission on Heart Disease, Stroke, and Cancer recommended only a few years ago that better medical care be brought to many areas that do not now have it. Obviously that is desirable, but there was not a word about the prevention of these diseases, the improvement of what might now be considered good health, or of the importance of good nutrition.) Fortunately, in the past year or so, the situation has changed for the better and we are beginning to think about preventing disease.

In the decade before World War II and for a few years thereafter, nutrition was one of the most active fields of research. This was undoubtedly stimulated by the medical profession's new awareness of widespread classical nutritional disease in the United States, particularly in the South but also in the North and by no means confined to the economically distressed. At the same time, the vitamins, which had been rather mysterious substances in which some medical scientists only half believed, were becoming clearly defined entities associated with clinically recognizable deficiency syndromes. Even their biochemical functions became apparent: for example, Warburg's yellow enzyme, important in cellular respiration, was shown to contain Vitamin B_2, riboflavin.

In an incredibly short time, the vitamins were purified, their chemical structures were defined, and means of synthesizing them were developed so that they were available in pure form for the treatment and prevention of deficiencies and for the fortification of certain key foods. Through the cooperation of biochemists, clinicians, manufacturers, and public health officials, acute vitamin deficiencies declined rapidly; by the end of World War II they were no longer a major cause of morbidity.

Then the science of nutrition suffered a curious fate. It seemed unable to perpetuate itself. No one was taking the place of Goldberger, Spies, Sydenstricker, Hart, Steenbock, Elvehjem, and Jolliffe, to mention only a few outstanding workers of the time. Why? Surely one could not conclude that because the field had made spectacular progress, nothing remained to be done. However, hearing some of the current generation rallying against the need for vitamin supplementation, one gains the impression that they do not really believe that a serious nutritional problem ever existed or can ever exist again. Surely the idea that the average "homo ineptus" eats an adequate diet simply because it is available is naivete unworthy of any scientist. Health education, which includes nutrition education, can be and should be vastly improved. True, the fortification of some of our common foods with various vitamins and minerals – white flour with three B-vitamins and the mineral iron, prepared cereals with various vitamins and minerals, margarines with vitamin A, milk with vitamin D, and many fruit-flavored drinks with vitamin C – has no doubt been important in lessening the classical nutritional deficiencies. While now only occasionally do obvious nutritional deficiencies force themselves on our attention, there is no satisfactory evidence that in their milder and more subtle forms they may not still be common. Furthermore, what evidence have we that we have obtained the ultimate in health through diet? Further food fortification may be the answer.

Perhaps it was thought that since the release of energy from food is a biochemical problem, nutrition would be adequately dealt with by the biochemists. True, much of biochemistry has nutritional significance, and biochemical research is constantly uncovering facts that bear on nutritional problems. Nevertheless, it is desirable that someone gather these facts and apply them to improved personal and public health and to practical clinical problems. After all, in a practical way, we would be "bad off" without engineers in spite of our competent physicists.

While vitamin deficiencies are no longer a pressing problem in the United States, we have other nutritional problems such as obesity, deficiency anemias, too much cholesterol and saturated fat, and possibly the whole problem of trace elements as exemplified by the lack of fluoride in our foods and water. Recent nutritional surveys in various parts of the United States indicated that 5% to 20% of the population may show various signs of mild vitamin and mineral deficiencies, so we may have more nutritional deficiencies than we are aware of.

We can reasonably well control blood glucose concentrations of diabetic patients and prevent death from diabetic ketoacidosis, but we still fail to prevent many of the serious sequelae, which are probably related primarily to caloric excess.

And how do we improve instruction in our medical schools so the physician of tomorrow will do a better job than the physician of today? There have been numerous conferences on the subject, with much verbiage, many generalities, but few positive results. The answer is very simple: employ a few qualified people to teach nutrition. Any medical school that received an endowed professorship of nutrition would soon be teaching nutrition. It is just that simple.

There is much in nutrition that relates directly and indirectly to health – to poor health if nutrition is poor, to good health if nutrition is good, and to better health if nutrition is the best. The purpose of this manual is to interest medical students, physicians, dentists, and other health professionals in the important role good nutrition plays in the health of their patients and themselves and to outline a few of the principles of modern nutrition; primarily, we hope to stimulate all to learn more about nutrition, to practice the best nutrition themselves, and to persuade their patients and friends to do likewise.

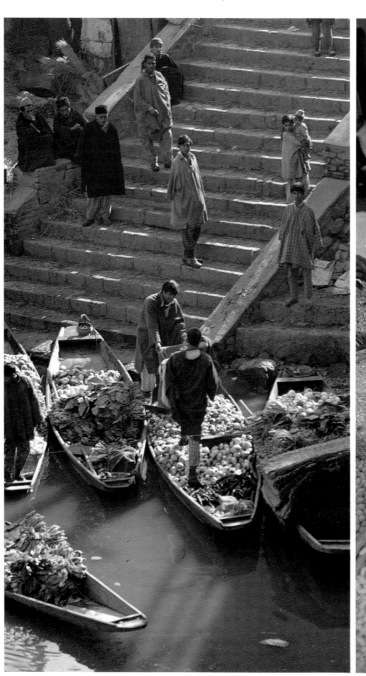
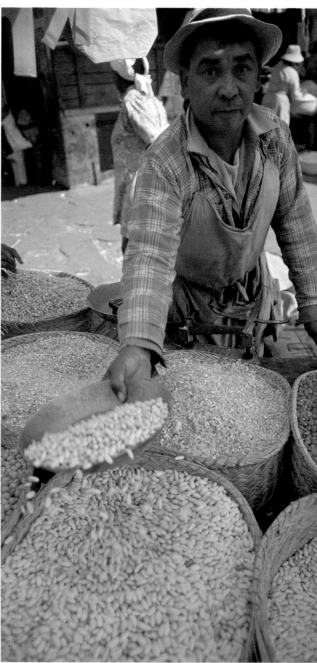

References

1. Ten-State Nutrition Survey 1968-1970, DHEW Pub No (HSM) 72-8134, Washington DC, US Govt Print Office, 1972.

2. *Recommended Dietary Allowances,* ed 7. Dietary Allowances Committee and Food and Nutrition Board, National Academy of Sciences, 1968.

3. *Recommended Dietary Allowances,* ed 9. Dietary Allowances Committee and Food and Nutrition Board, National Academy of Sciences, 1980 (in press).

4. Report of Inter-Society Commission for Heart Disease Resources. *Circulation 42*:A55-A95, 1970.

5. Leren P: The Oslo diet-heart study: Eleven year report. *Circulation 42:* 935-942, 1970.

6. Fredrickson DS, Levy RI, Lees RS: Fat transport in lipoproteins – An integrated approach to mechanisms and disorders. *N Engl J Med 276:* 34-42, 94-103, 148-156, 215-225, 273-281, 1967.

7. Miller GJ, Miller NE: Plasma-high-density-lipoprotein concentration and development of ischaemic heart disease. *Lancet I:*16-19, 1975.

8. Bierman EL, Albrink MJ, Arky RA, Connor WE, Dayton S, Spritz N, Steinberg D (Committee of Food and Nutrition of the American Diabetes Association): Special report: Principles of nutrition for patients with diabetes mellitus. *Diabetes 20:*633-634, 1971.

9. West KM: Prevention and therapy of diabetes mellitus, in Hegsted DM, Chichester CO, Darby WJ, McNutt KW, Stalvey RM, Stotz EH (eds): *Present Knowledge in Nutrition,* ed 4. New York, The Nutrition Foundation, 1976, pp 356-364.

10. Weinsier RL, Seeman A, Herrera MG: Diet therapy of diabetes. Description of a successful methodologic approach to gaining diet adherence. *Diabetes 23:*669-673, 1974.

11. Shaw JH, Sweeney EA: Nutrition in relation to dental medicine, in Goodhart RS, Shils ME (eds): *Modern Nutrition in Health and Disease: Dietotherapy,* ed 5. Philadelphia, Lea & Febiger, 1973, pp 733-769.

12. Erickson JD, David J: Mortality in selected cities with fluoridated and nonfluoridated water supplies. *N Engl J Med 298:*1112-1116, 1978.

13. The attack on fluoridation. *Consumer Reports,* July 392-396, August 480-482, 1978.

14. Ast DB, Cons NC, Pollard ST, Garfinkel J: Time and cost factors to provide regular, periodic dental care for children in a fluoridated and nonfluoridated area: Final report. *J Am Dent Assoc 80:*770-776, 1970.

15. Bernstein DS, Sadowsky N, Hegsted DM, Guri CD, Stare FJ: Prevalence of osteoporosis in high- and low-fluoride areas in North Dakota. *JAMA 198:* 499-504, 1966.

16. Bernstein DS, Cohen P: Use of sodium fluoride in the treatment of osteoporosis. *J Clin Endocrinol 27:*197-210, 1967.

17. Leone NC, Stevenson CA, Besse B, Hawes LF, Dawber TR: The effects of the absorption of fluoride. *Arch Indust Health 21:*326-327, 1960.

18. Hegsted DM: Nutrition, bone, and calcified tissue. *J Am Diet Assoc 50:* 105-111, 1967.

19. A symposium sponsored by the American Cancer Society and the National Cancer Institute on Nutrition in the Causation of Cancer. *Cancer Research 35* (No 11 pt 2):3231-3543, 1975.

20. Control of nutritional anaemia with special reference to iron deficiency: Report of an IAEA/USAID/WHO joint meeting. *WHO Tech Rep Ser 580:* 1-75, 1975.

21. Sayers MH, Lynch SR, Charlton RW, Walker RB, Maye TF: The fortification of common salt with ascorbic acid and iron. *Br J Haematol 28:*483-495, 1974.

22. Latham MC: Adapted from *Human Nutrition in Tropical Africa* (ed 8), Food and Nutrition Series: No 11. Rome, FAO, 1965.

23. Whitehead RG: Hydroxyproline creatinine ratio as an index of nutritional status and rate of growth. *Lancet II:*567-570, 1965.

24. Gomez F, Galvan RR, Frenk S, Munoz JC, Chavez R, Vazchez J: Mortality in second and third degree malnutrition. *J Trop Pediatr 2:*77-83, 1956.

25. Latham MC: Pre- and post-kwashiorkor and marasmus, in McCance RA, Widdowson EM (eds): *Calorie Deficiencies and Protein Deficiencies.* London, J and A Churchill Ltd, 1968, pp 23-30.

26. Jelliffe DB: *The Assessment of the Nutritional Status of the Community.* Geneva, WHO, 1966.

27. Pollitt E, Thomson C: Protein-calorie malnutrition and behavior: A view from psychology, in Wurtman RJ, Wurtman JJ (eds): *Nutrition and the Brain,* vol 2. New York, Raven Press, 1977, pp 261-306.

28. Winick M, Noble A: Cellular response in rats during malnutrition at various ages. *J Nutr 89:*300-306, 1966.

29. Lubchenco LO: *The High Risk Infant.* Philadelphia, WB Saunders, 1976.

30. Stoch MB, Smythe PM: The effect of undernutrition during infancy and subsequent brain growth and intellectual development. *S Afr Med J 41:* 1027-1030, 1967.

31. Nutrition and infection: Report of a WHO expert committee. *WHO Tech Rep Ser 314:*1-30, 1965.

32. Keusch GT, Katz M (eds): Symposium: Effective interventions to reduce infection in malnourished populations. *Am J Clin Nutr 31:*2035-2126, 2202-2356, 1978.

33. Pitkin RM: Obstetrics and gynecology, in Schneider HA, Anderson CE, Coursin DB (eds): *Nutritional Support of Medical Practice,* Hagerstown MD, Harper & Row, 1977, pp 407-421.

34. Vitamin A deficiency and xerophthalmia: Report of a joint WHO/USAID meeting. *WHO Tech Rep Ser 590:*1-88, 1976.

35. Smith FR, Goodman DS, Zaklama MS: Serum vitamin A, retinol-binding protein, and prealbumin concentrations in protein-calorie malnutrition. I. A functional defect in hepatic retinol release. *Am J Clin Nutr 26:*973-981, 1973.

36. Victor M, Adams RD: On the etiology of the alcoholic neurologic diseases. *Am J Clin Nutr 9:*379-397, 1961.

37. Latham MC: Present knowledge of thiamin, in Hegsted DM, Chichester CO, Darby WJ, McNutt KW, Stalvey RM, Stotz EH (eds): *Present Knowledge in Nutrition*, ed 3. New York, The Nutrition Foundation, 1967, pp 55-60.

38. Ingbar SH, Woeber KA: Disease of the thyroid, in Thorn GW, Adams RD, Braunwald E, Isselbacher KJ, Petersdorf RG (eds): *Harrison's Principles of Internal Medicine*, ed 8. New York, McGraw-Hill, 1977, chap 92, pp 501-519.

39. Endemic Goitre. *WHO Monograph Series 44*:1-471, 1960.

40. Irwin MD, Hegsted DM: A conspectus of research on amino acid requirements in man. *J Nutr 101*:539-566, 1971.

41. Hayes KC: A review on the biological function of taurine. *Nutr Rev 34*: 161-165,1976.

42. el Lozy M, Hegsted DM: Calculation of the amino acid requirements of children at different ages by the factorial method. *Am J Clin Nutr 28*:1052-1054, 1975.

43. Adibi SA: Intestinal phase of protein assimilation in man. *Am J Clin Nutr 29*:205-215, 1976.

44. Baker SJ, DeMaeyer EM: Nutritional Anemia: Its understanding and control with special reference to the work of the World Health Organization. *Am J Clin Nutr 32*:368-417, 1979.

45. Monsen ER, Hallberg L, Layrine M, Hegsted DM, Cook JD, Mertz W, Finch CA: Estimation of available dietary iron. *Am J Clin Nutr 31*:134-141,1978.

46. Frenchman R, Johnston FA: Relation of menstrual losses to iron requirement. *J Am Diet Assoc 25*:217-220, 1949.

47. MacPhail AP, Simon MO, Torrance JD, Charlton RW, Bothwell TH, Isaacson C. Changing patterns of dietary iron overload in black South Africans. *Am J Clin Nutr 32*:1272-1278, 1979.

48. Calcium requirements: Report of an FAO/WHO expert group. *WHO Tech Rep Ser 230*:1-54, 1962.

49. Cavalieri RR: Iodine, in Goodhart RS, Shils ME (eds): *Modern Nutrition in Health and Disease: Dietotherapy*, ed 5. Philadelphia, Lea & Febiger, 1973, pp 362-371.

50. Gaiton E, Meyer JD, Merino H: Environmental goitrogens in Colombia, in Dunn JT, Medeiros-Neto GA (eds): *Endemic Goiter and Cretinism: Continuing Threats to World Health*. Washington, PAHO, 1974, pp 107-117.

51. Schwarz K, Milne DB: Fluoride requirements for growth in the rat. *Bioinorganic Chem 1*:331-338, 1972.

52. Messer HH, Armstrong WD, Singer L: Fertility impairment in mice on a low fluoride intake. *Science 177*:893-894, 1972.

53. Singh A, Malhotra KC, Singh BM, Mattur OC: Endemic fluorosis. *Indian J Med Sc 20*:569-574, 1966.

54. Latham MC, Grech P: The effects of excessive fluoride intake. *Am J Pub Health 57*:651-660, 1956.

55. Darrow DC, Pratt EL, Flett T, Gamble AH, Wiese HF: Disturbances in water and electrolytes in infantile diarrhea. *Pediatrics 3*:129-156, 1949.

56. Schroeder HA, Nason AP, Tipton IH: Essential metals in man: Magnesium. *J Chronic Dis 21*:815-841, 1969.

57. Vallee BE, Wacker WEC, Ulmer DD: The magnesium deficiency tetany syndrome in man. *N Engl J Med 262*:155-161, 1960.

58. Wacker WEC, Moore FD, Ulmer DO, Vallee BE: Normocalcemic magnesium deficiency tetany. *JAMA 180*:161, 1962.

59. Montgomery RD: Magnesium metabolism in infantile protein malnutrition. *Lancet II*:74-75, 1960.

60. Patwardhan VN: Hypervitaminosis A and epidemiology of xerophthalmia. *Am J Clin Nutr 22*:1106-1118, 1969.

61. Sauberlich HE, Dowdy RP, Skala TH: *Laboratory Tests for the Assessment of Nutritional Status*. Cleveland, CRC Press, 1974.

62. Bergen SS Jr, Roels OA: Hypervitaminosis A: Report of a case. *Amer J Clin Nutr 16*:265-269, 1965.

63. Eijkman C: Eine Beriberiatinliche Krankheit der Huehnes. *Virchow's Arch Path Anat 148*:523, 1897; and Ein Versuch zur Bekamtfung der Beriberi. *Virchow's Arch Path Anat 149*:183, 1897.

64. Grijns G: Beriberi on rijstveeding. *Tidjsch V Nederl Indie 41*:3, 1901.

65. McCollum EV, Kennedy C: The dietary factors operating in the production of polyneuritis. *J Biol Chem 24*:491-502, 1916.

66. Brin M: Thiamine deficiency and erythrocyte metabolism. *Am J Clin Nutr 12*:107-116, 1963.

67. Tanphaichitr V: Thiamin, in Hegsted DM, Chichester CO, Darby WJ, McNutt KW, Stalvey RM, Stotz EH (eds): *Present Knowledge in Nutrition*, ed 4. New York, The Nutrition Foundation, 1976, pp 141-148.

68. Rivlin RS: Riboflavin metabolism. *N Engl J Med 283*:463-472, 1970.

69. Anon: Forms of bound niacin in wheat. *Nutr Reviews 32*:124-125, 1974.

70. Darby WJ, NcNutt KW, Todhunter EH: Niacin, in Hegsted DM, Chichester CO, Darby WJ, McNutt KW, Stalvey RM, Stotz EH (eds): *Present Knowledge in Nutrition*, ed 4. New York, The Nutrition Foundation, 1976, pp 162-174.

71. Gershoff SN, Prien EL: Excretion of urinary metabolites in calcium oxalate urolithiasis. *Am J Clin Nutr 8*:812-816, 1960.

72. Cornish HH: The role of vitamin B_6 in the toxicity of hydrazines. *Ann NY Acad Sci 166*:136-145, 1969.

73. Dempsey WB: Vitamin B_6 and pregnancy, in Food and Nutrition Board (eds): *Human Vitamin B_6 Requirements*. Washington, NAS-NRC, 1978, pp 202-209.

74. Donald EA, Bosse TR: The vitamin B_6 requirement of oral contraceptive users. II. Assessment by tryptophan metabolites, vitamin B_6 and pyridoxic acid levels in urine. *Am J Clin Nutr 32*: 1024-1037, 1979.

75. Rose DP: Oral contraceptives and vitamin B_6, in Food and Nutrition Board (eds): *Human Vitamin B_6 Requirements*. Washington, NAS-NRC, 1978, pp 193-201.

76. Hodges RE, Bean WB, Ohlson Margaret A, Bleiler Roberta: Human pantothenic acid deficiency produced by omega-methyl pathothenic acid. *J Clin Invest 38*:1421-1425, 1959.

77. Silber R, Moldow CF: The biochemistry of B_{12}-mediated reactions in man. *Am J Med 48*:549-554, 1970.

78. Castle WB: Current concepts of pernicious anemia. *Am J Med 48*:541-548, 1970.

79. Wokes F, Badenoch J, Sinclair HM: Human dietary deficiency of vitamin B_{12}. *Am J Clin Nutr 3*:375-382, 1955.

80. Luhby AL, Cooperman JM: Folic acid deficiency in man and its interrelationship with vitamin B_{12} metabolism. *Adv Metab Disord 1*:263-336, 1964.

81. Herbert V: Biochemical and hematologic lesions in folic acid deficiency. *Am J Clin Nutr 20*:562-572, 1967.

82. Vilter RW, Will JJ, Wright T, Pullman D: Interrelationships of vitamin B_{12}, folic acid and ascorbic acid in the megaloblastic anemias. *Am J Clin Nutr 12*: 130-144, 1963.

83. Stocksted ELR: Regulation of folate metabolism by vitamin B_{12}, in Food and Nutrition Board (eds): *Folic Acid Biochemistry and Physiology in Relation to the Human Nutritional Requirement.* Washington, NAS-NRC, 1977, pp 122-135.

84. Herbert V: Experimental nutritional folate deficiency in man. *Tr Assoc Am Phys 75*:307-320, 1962.

85. Herbert V, Jacob E: Destruction of vitamin B_{12} by ascorbic acid. *JAMA 230*:241-242, 1974.

86. Hines JD: (letter) Ascorbic acid and vitamin B_{12} deficiency. *JAMA 234*: 24, 1975.

87. Ohmdahl JL, DeLuca HF: Regulation of vitamin D metabolism and function. *Physiol Rev 53*:327-372, 1973.

88. Haussler MR: Vitamin D, in Hegsted DM, Chichester CO, Darby WJ, McNutt KW, Stalvey RM, Stotz EH (eds): *Present Knowledge in Nutrition,* ed 4. New York, The Nutrition Foundation, 1976, pp 82-97.

89. Report of the Committee of Nutrition, American Academy of Pediatrics. *Pediatrics 31*:512, 1963.

90. Moore CV: Iron, in Goodhart RS, Shils ME (eds): *Modern Nutrition in Health and Disease: Dietotherapy,* ed 5. Philadelphia, Lea & Febiger, 1973, pp 297-323.

91. Latham MC: Nutrition and infection in national development. *Science 188*:561-565, 1975.

92. Kapikian AZ, Kim HW, Wyatt RG, Cline WL, Arrobio JO, Brandt CD, Rodriguez MD, Sack DA, Channock RM, Parrott RH: Human reovirus-like agent as the major pathogen associated with 'winter' gastroenteritis in hospitalized infants and young children. *N Engl J Med 294*:965-972, 1976.

93. Neumann CG, Lawlor GJ Jr, Stiehm ER: Immunologic responses in malnourished children. *Am J Clin Nutr 28*:80-104, 1975.

94. Hambraeus L: Proprietary milk versus human breast milk in infant feeding: A critical appraisal from the nutritional point of view. *Pediatr Clin North Am 24*:17-36, 1977.

95. Latham MC: Regulation and education: Strategies for solving the bottle feeding problem, in Greiner T (ed): *Cornell International Nutrition Monograph No. 4.* Ithaca NY, Cornell Univ, 1977, pp i-xiv.

96. Greiner T: The promotion of bottle feeding by multinational corporations: How advertising and the health professions have contributed. *Cornell International Nutrition Monograph No 2.* Ithaca NY, Cornell Univ, 1975.

97. Butterworth CE Jr: (Editorial) Malnutrition in the hospital. *JAMA 230*: 879, 1974.

98. Blackburn GL, Bistrian BR, Curative nutrition: Protein-calorie management, in Schnieder HA, Anderson CE, Courier DB (eds): *Nutritional Support of Medical Practice.* New York, Hagerstown MD, Harper & Row, 1977, pp 80-100.

99. Holzel A: Sugar malabsorption due to deficiencies of disaccharidase activities and monosaccharide transport. *Arch Dis Child 42*:341-352, 1967.

100. Crane RK: A perspective of digestive-absorptive function. *Am J Clin Nutr 22*:242-249, 1969.

101. Bayless TM, Christopher NL: Disaccharidase deficiency. *Am J Clin Nutr 22*:181-190, 1969.

102. Protein Advisory Group of the United Nations: Milk intolerance–nutritional implications, Document 1.27/9, 1972.

103. Stephenson LS, Latham MC: Lactose intolerance and milk consumption: The relation of tolerance to symptoms. *Am J Clin Nutr 27*:296-303, 1974.

104. Burkitt DP: Western civilization, diet and disease. *Drug Therapy*:51-62, January 1974.

105. Painter NS, Almeida AZ, Colebourne KW: Unprocessed bran in treatment of diverticular disease of the colon. *Brit Med J 2*:137-140, 1972.

106. Marabou Symposium, Food and Fibre, Supplement No.14, Naringsforskning, argang 20, 1-72, 1976.

107. Symposium on Role of Dietary Fiber in Health. *Am J Clin Nutr 31*(suppl); S1-S291, October, 1978.

108. Hartshorn EA: Food and drug interactions. *J Am Diet Assoc 70*:15, 1977.

109. Barn TK: Interaction of drugs and nutrition. *J Human Nutr 31*:449, 1977.

110. Dietary Goals for the United States, Senate Select Committee on Nutrition, 1977.

111. Nutrition Today: Twenty commentaries. *Nutrition Today 12* (6):10-13, 20-27, 1977.

112. Nutrition Today: Additional commentaries. *Nutrition Today 13 (1)*30-32,1978.

113. (Revised) Dietary Goals for the United States. Senate Select Committee on Nutrition, 1978.

114. Symposium: Report of the task force on the evidence relating six dietary factors to the nation's health. *Am J Clin Nutr 32*:2621-2748, 1979.

Table of sodium, potassium, and magnesium content of selected foods[1]

Food, amount	(grams)	Na (mg)	K (mg)	Mg (mg)
Apple: raw, 1 med	150	2	165	8
Apricot: raw, 1 med	40	Trace	112	5
Avocado: raw, cubed, ¼ cup	36	1	217	16
Bacon:				
fried or broiled, 2 slices	14	143	33	4
Canadian, fried or broiled, 2 oz	57	1456	246	14
Banana: raw, 1 med	150	2	555	50
Beans: baked (no pork), 1 cup	187	632	501	69
Beef: lean, cooked, 4 oz	113	68	418	33
Bread:				
Rye, regular, 1 slice	23	128	33	10
Rye, unsalted, 1 slice	23	7	26	10
White, enriched, 1 slice	23	117	24	5
White, unsalted, 1 slice	23	7	41	5
Whole wheat, 1 slice	23	121	63	18
Whole wheat, unsalted, 1 slice	23	7	53	18
Butter:				
Regular, 1 pat	7	69	2	Trace
Unsalted, 1 pat	7	Trace	2	Trace
Cabbage: raw, shredded, 1 cup	73	15	170	10
Cantaloupe or honey dew:				
½ whole, med	385	46	966	62
Carrots: raw, 1 med	50	24	171	12
Cauliflower: raw, 1 cup	104	14	307	25
Celery: raw, 1 stalk	40	50	136	9
Cereals:				
Cornflakes, 1 cup	28	281	34	5
Puffed rice, unsalted, 1 cup	14	Trace	14	—
Puffed wheat, unsalted, 1 cup	14	Trace	48	—
Cheese:				
Cheddar, 1 oz	28	196	23	13
Cottage, creamed, 1 cup	225	515	191	—
Cherries: sweet or sour, 1 cup	130	3	248	10-18
Chicken: cooked:				
White meat, 4 oz	113	72	498	22
Dark meat, 4 oz	113	97	363	—
Chocolate: bitter, 1 oz	28	1	232	82
Chocolate syrup: 1 tbsp	20	10	56	13
Coffee: instant dry powder, 1 tsp	1	1	33	5
Corn, sweet:				
Cooked, 1 ear	100	15	165	—
Canned, 1 cup	169	399	164	32
Crackers:				
Graham, 1 square	7	47	27	4
Soda, 2″ square, 2 squares	8	88	10	2
Egg: whole, 1 med	50	61	65	6
Fish:				
Cod, broiled, 4 oz	113	124	460	32
Haddock, fried, 4 oz	113	200	393	27
Halibut, broiled, 4 oz	113	151	593	—
Tuna, water packed, ½ cup	115	47	321	—
Grapefruit: sections, 1 cup	194	2	262	23
Grapes: slip skin, 1 cup	153	5	242	20
Honey: strained, 1 tbsp	21	1	11	1
Ice cream: vanilla, 1 scoop	71	45	129	10
Jam: jelly (assorted), 1 tbsp	20	3	16	2
Lamb: any cut, broiled or roasted, 4 oz	113	79	328	21
Lettuce: iceberg, 1/6 head	43	4	75	5
Lobster: cooked, 4 oz	113	237	203	25
Macaroni: plain, cooked, 1 cup	140	1	85	25
Margarine:				
Regular, 1 pat	7	69	2	—
Unsalted, 1 pat	7	Trace	1	—
Milk:				
Whole, 3.7% fat, 1 cup	244	122	351	32
Skim, 1 cup	246	123	354	34
Evaporated, unsweetened, 1 cup	252	297	764	63
Noodles: cooked, 1 cup	160	3	70	—
Olives:				
Green, 1 med	6	144	3	1
Ripe, 1 med	6	45	2	—

Food, amount	(grams)	Na (mg)	K (mg)	Mg (mg)
Onions: mature, raw, 1 slice	17	2	27	2
Orange: 1 med	180	2	360	20
Orange juice: 1 cup	249	3	498	27
Pancakes: from mix, 1 med	45	203	70	—
Peaches: raw, 1 med	114	1	230	11
Peanuts: roasted, unsalted, 1 oz	28	1	196	49
Peanut butter: 1 tbsp	16	97	104	28
Pears: raw, 1 small	75	2	98	5
Peas:				
Canned, regular, 1 cup	160	378	154	32
Frozen, 1 cup	160	184	216	38
Canned, low sodium, 1 cup	160	5	154	38
Pickles:				
Dill, 1 med, whole	100	1428	200	12
Sweet, 1 small, whole	20	105	—	Trace
Pineapple:				
Raw, diced, 1 cup	140	1	204	18
Canned, heavy syrup, 2 slices	122	1	117	10
Plums: raw, 1 med	60	Trace	102	5
Pork:				
All cuts, lean, cooked, 4 oz	113	74	441	26
Ham, cured, cooked, 4 oz	113	1051	368	19
Sausage, cooked, 1 link	20	192	54	3
Potatoes:				
Peeled, boiled, unsalted, 1 med	122	2	348	27
French fried, unsalted, 10 pieces	57	3	486	14
Mashed, milk added, 1 cup	195	587	509	23
Potato chips, 10 med	20	200*	226	—
Pretzels: 1 med	20	336	26	—
Pumpkin: canned, unsalted, 1 cup	228	5	547	27
Raisins: uncooked, 1 snack pack	18	5	137	6
Rice:				
Cooked, regular, salted, 1 cup	193	722	54	15
Cooked, unsalted, 1 cup	193	4	54	15
Salad dressings:				
French, 1 tbsp	15	206	12	2
Italian, 1 tbsp	15	314	2	—
Mayonnaise, 1 tbsp	15	90	5	Trace
Russian, 1 tbsp	15	130	24	—
Shrimp: cooked, 4 oz	113	210	259	58
Syrup: maple, 1 tbsp	20	2	35	2
Spinach: cooked, 1 cup	180	90	583	113
Squash: summer, cooked, unsalted, 1 cup	136	1	192	22
Strawberries: raw, 1 cup	144	1	236	17
Sweet potato: baked, 1	110	13	330	34
Tangerine: raw, 1 med	114	1	144	—
Tomato: raw, 1 med	120	4	293	17
Tomato juice:				
Canned, 1 cup	242	484	549	24
Canned, low sodium, 1 cup	242	7	549	24
Tomato catsup:				
Regular, 1 tbsp	17	228	63	4
Low sodium, 1 tbsp	17	1-6	63	4
Turkey: roasted, 4 oz	113	147	415	32
Veal: all cuts, cooked, 3 oz	85	68	425	15
Watermelon:				
1/16 med. melon, 1–4″ x 8″ wedge	925	9	925	74
Yogurt: 1 cup	244	124	349	—

* Varies greatly according to amount of added salt

– denotes unknown

1 Mitchell HS, et al (eds): Nutrition in Health and Disease, ed 16. New York, Lippincott, 1976.

Table of Nutritive Values of the Edible Part of Foods[1]

(Dashes show that no basis could be found for computing a value although there was some reason to believe that a measurable amount of the constituent might be present.)

Food, approximate measure, and weight	Water %	Calories	Protein	Fat (Total lipid)	Saturated	Oleic	Linoleic	Carbohydrate	Calcium	Phosphorus	Iron	Vitamin A	Thiamine	Riboflavin	Niacin	Ascorbic acid
			gm	gm	gm	gm	gm	gm	mg	mg	mg	IU	mg	mg	mg	mg
MILK, CREAM, CHEESE; RELATED PRODUCTS																
Milk, cows':																
Fluid, whole (3.3% fat), 1 cup (244 gm)	88	150	8	8	5.1	2.1	.2	11	291	228	.1	310	.09	.40	.2	2
Fluid, nonfat (skim), 1 cup (245 gm)	91	85	8	tr	.3	.1	tr	12	302	247	.1	500	.09	.37	.2	2
Cheese:																
Cheddar, 1 oz slice (28 gm)	37	115	7	9	6.1	2.1	.2	tr	204	145	.2	300	.01	.11	tr	0
Cottage, creamed, 1 cup (225 gm)	79	235	28	10	6.4	2.4	.2	6	135	297	.3	370	.05	.37	.3	tr
Ice cream, vanilla, 1 cup (133 gm)	61	270	5	14	8.9	3.6	.3	32	176	134	.1	540	.05	.33	.1	1
EGGS																
Raw, whole, 1 med (50 gm)	75	80	6	6	1.7	2.0	.6	1	28	90	1.0	260	.04	.15	tr	0
MEAT, POULTRY, FISH, SHELLFISH; RELATED PRODUCTS																
Beef, cooked:																
Roast, relatively lean such as heel of round																
Lean and fat, 3 oz (85 gm)	62	165	25	7	2.8	2.7	.2	0	11	208	3.2	10	.06	.19	4.5	—
Lean only, 2.9 oz (78 gm)	65	125	24	3	1.2	1.0	.1	0	10	199	3.0	tr	.06	.18	4.3	—
Steak, relatively fat–sirloin, broiled																
Lean and fat, 3 oz (85 gm)	44	330	20	27	11.3	11.1	.6	0	9	162	2.5	50	.05	.15	4.0	—
Lean only, 2 oz (51 gm)	59	115	18	4	1.8	1.6	.2	0	7	146	2.2	10	.05	.14	3.6	—
Ground beef, broiled																
Lean with 10% fat, 3 oz (85 gm)	60	185	23	10	4.0	3.9	.3	0	10	196	3.0	20	.08	.20	5.1	—
Lean with 21% fat, 2.9 oz (82 gm)	54	235	20	17	7.0	6.7	.4	0	9	159	2.6	30	.07	.17	4.4	—
Corned beef, canned, 3 oz (85 gm)	59	185	22	10	4.9	4.5	.2	0	17	90	3.7	—	.01	.20	2.9	—
Pork, cooked:																
Ham, baked																
Lean and fat, 3 oz (85 gm)	54	245	18	19	6.8	7.9	1.7	0	8	146	2.2	0	.40	.15	3.1	0
Roast pork																
Lean and fat, 3 oz (85 gm)	46	310	21	24	8.7	10.2	2.2	0	9	218	2.7	0	.78	.22	4.8	—
Lean only, 2.4 oz (68 gm)	55	175	20	10	3.5	4.1	.8	0	9	211	2.6	0	.73	.21	4.4	—
(visible fat removed at table)																
Loin chop, lean only, 2 oz (56 gm)	53	150	17	9	3.1	??	0.8	0	7	181	2.2	0	.63	.18	3.8	—
Lamb, cooked:																
Roast leg, lean only, 2.5 oz (71 gm)	62	130	20	5	2.1	1.8	.2	0	9	169	1.4	—	.12	.21	4.4	—
Veal, cooked:																
Cutlet, medium fat, 3 oz (85 gm)	60	185	23	9	4.0	3.4	.4	0	9	196	2.7	—	.06	.21	4.6	—
Chicken, cooked:																
Half broiler, bones removed, 6.2 oz (176 gm)	71	240	42	7	2.2	2.5	1.3	0	16	355	3.0	160	.09	.34	15.5	—
Fish, cooked:																
Fish baked with butter or margarine, 3 oz (85 gm)	68	135	22	4	—	—	—	0	25	244	0.6	40	.09	.08	1.6	—
Tuna, packed in oil, drained solids 3 oz (85 gm)	61	170	24	7	1.7	1.7	.7	0	7	199	1.6	70	.04	.10	10.1	—
Shrimp, canned meat, 3 oz (85 gm)	70	100	21	1	.1	.1	tr	1	98	224	2.6	50	.01	.03	1.5	—
Meat and meat products:																
Bacon, broiled or fried, 2 slices (15 gm)	8	85	4	8	2.5	3.7	.7	tr	2	34	.5	0	.08	.05	.8	—
Frankfurter, cooked, 1 (56 gm)	57	170	7	15	5.6	6.5	1.2	1	3	57	.8	—	.08	.11	1.4	—
Liver, beef, fried, 3 oz (85 gm)	56	195	22	9	2.5	3.5	.9	5	9	405	7.5	45,390	.22	3.56	14.0	23
VEGETABLES AND VEGETABLE PRODUCTS																
Asparagus:																
Cooked, 1 cup (145 gm)	94	30	3	tr	—	—	—	5	30	73	0.9	1,310	.23	.26	2.0	38
Beans:																
Lima, frozen, cooked, 1 cup (170 gm)	74	170	10	tr	—	—	—	32	34	153	2.9	390	.12	.09	1.7	29
Snap, green, cooked, 1 cup (125 gm)	92	30	2	tr	—	—	—	7	63	46	.8	680	.09	.11	.6	15
Baked, with tomato sauce, pork, 1 cup (255 gm)	71	310	16	7	2.4	2.8	.6	48	138	235	4.6	330	.20	.08	1.5	5
Beets:																
Cooked, sliced, 1 cup (170 gm)	91	55	2	tr	—	—	—	12	24	39	.9	30	.05	.07	.5	10
Broccoli:																
Cooked, 1 cup (155 gm)	91	40	5	tr	—	—	—	7	136	96	1.2	3,880	.14	.31	1.2	140

tr = trace

1. These values are taken from "Nutritive Value of Foods," Home and Garden Bulletin, No. 72, Agricultural Research Service, revised 1978, and represent only a small portion of the total foods given in the Bulletin. The complete table is available from Superintendent of Documents, U.S. Government Printing Office, Washington, D.C. for $1.05– Stock # 001-000-03667-0.

Table of Nutritive Values of the Edible Part of Foods

(Dashes show that no basis could be found for computing a value although there was some reason to believe that a measurable amount of the constituent might be present.)

Food, approximate measure, and weight	Water %	Cal-ories	Pro-tein	Fat (Total lipid)	Fatty Acids Satu-rated	Fatty Acids Unsaturated Oleic	Fatty Acids Unsaturated Lino-leic	Car-bohy-drate	Cal-cium	Phos-pho-rus	Iron	Vitamin A	Thia-mine	Ribo-flavin	Nia-cin	Ascor-bic acid
			gm	gm	gm	gm	gm	gm	mg	mg	mg	IU	mg	mg	mg	mg
Cabbage:																
Shredded, raw, 1 cup (90 gm)	92	20	1	tr	—	—	—	5	44	26	.4	120	.05	.05	.3	42
Cooked, 1 cup (145 gm)	94	30	2	tr	—	—	—	6	64	29	.4	190	.06	.06	.4	48
Carrots:																
Cooked, sliced, 1 cup (155 gm)	91	50	1	tr	—	—	—	11	51	48	.9	16,280	.08	.08	.8	9
Cauliflower:																
Cooked, 1 cup (125 gm)	93	30	3	tr	—	—	—	5	26	53	.9	80	.11	.10	.8	69
Celery:																
Raw, 1 stalk (40 gm)	94	5	tr	tr	—	—	—	2	16	11	.1	110	.01	.01	.1	4
Corn, sweet:																
Cooked, 1 ear (140 gm)	74	70	2	1	—	—	—	16	2	69	.5	310	.09	.08	1.1	7
Canned, 1 cup (165 gm)	76	140	4	1	—	—	—	33	8	81	.8	580	.05	.08	1.5	7
Cucumbers:																
Raw, without peel, 9 thin slices (28 gm)	96	5	tr	tr	—	—	—	1	5	5	.01	tr	.01	.01	.1	3
Lettuce:																
Chopped, 1 cup (55 gm)	96	5	tr	tr	—	—	—	2	11	12	.3	180	.03	.03	.2	3
Mushrooms:																
Raw, sliced, 1 cup (70 gm)	90	20	2	tr	—	—	—	3	4	81	.6	tr	.07	.32	2.9	2
Onions:																
Cooked, 1 cup (210 gm)	92	60	3	tr	—	—	—	14	50	61	.8	tr	.06	.06	.4	15
Parsnips:																
Cooked, 1 cup (105 gm)	82	100	2	1	—	—	—	23	70	96	.9	50	.11	.12	.2	16
Peas:																
Canned, 1 cup (170 gm)	77	150	8	1	—	—	—	29	44	129	3.2	1,170	.15	.10	1.4	14
Peppers:																
Sweet, raw, 1 pod (74 gm)	93	15	1	tr	—	—	—	4	7	16	.5	310	.06	.06	.4	94
Potatoes, medium, cooked:																
Baked, peeled, 1 potato (156 gm)	75	145	4	tr	—	—	—	33	14	101	1.1	tr	.15	.07	2.7	31
Peeled, boiled, 1 potato (135 gm)	83	90	3	tr	—	—	—	20	8	57	.7	tr	.12	.05	1.6	22
French-fried, 10 pieces (50 gm)	45	135	2	7	1.7	1.2	3.3	18	8	56	.7	tr	.07	.04	1.6	11
Mashed with milk and butter, 1 cup (210 gm)	80	195	4	9	5.6	2.3	0.2	26	50	101	0.8	360	.17	.11	2.1	19
Potato chips, 10 chips (20 gm)	2	115	1	8	2.1	1.4	4.0	10	8	28	.4	tr	.04	.01	1.0	3
Pumpkin:																
Canned, 1 cup (245 gm)	90	80	2	1	—	—	—	19	61	64	1.0	15,680	.07	.12	1.5	12
Radishes:																
4 small (18 gm)	95	5	tr	tr	—	—	—	1	5	6	.2	tr	.01	.01	.1	5
Sauerkraut, canned:																
Solids and liquid, 1 cup (235 gm)	93	40	2	tr	—	—	—	9	85	42	1.2	120	.07	.09	.5	33
Spinach:																
Cooked, 1 cup (180 gm)	92	40	5	1	—	—	—	6	167	68	4.0	14,580	.13	.25	.9	50
Squash, summer:																
Cooked, diced, 1 cup (210 gm)	96	30	2	tr	—	—	—	7	53	53	.8	820	.11	.17	1.7	21
Sweet potatoes:																
Baked, peeled, 1 potato (114 gm)	64	160	2	1	—	—	—	37	46	66	1.0	9,230	.10	.08	.8	25
Tomatoes:																
Raw, 1 tomato (135 gm)	94	25	1	tr	—	—	—	6	16	33	.6	1,110	.07	.05	.9	28
Tomato juice:																
Canned, 1 cup (243 gm)	94	45	2	tr	—	—	—	10	17	44	2.2	1,940	.12	.07	1.9	39
Tomato catsup:																
1 tbsp (15 gm)	69	15	tr	tr	—	—	—	4	3	8	.1	210	.01	.01	.2	2
Turnips:																
Cooked, diced, 1 cup (155 gm)	94	35	1	tr	—	—	—	8	54	37	.6	tr	.06	.08	.5	34

FRUITS AND FRUIT PRODUCTS

Food, approximate measure, and weight	Water %	Cal-ories	Pro-tein	Fat (Total lipid)	Satu-rated	Oleic	Lino-leic	Car-bohy-drate	Cal-cium	Phos-pho-rus	Iron	Vitamin A	Thia-mine	Ribo-flavin	Nia-cin	Ascor-bic acid
Apples:																
Raw, 1 med (138 gm)	84	80	tr	1	—	—	—	20	10	14	.4	120	.04	.03	.1	6
Apple juice: 1 cup (248 gm)	88	120	tr	tr	—	—	—	30	15	22	1.5	—	.02	.05	.2	2

tr = trace

Table of Nutritive Values of the Edible Part of Foods

(Dashes show that no basis could be found for computing a value although there was some reason to believe that a measurable amount of the constituent might be present.)

Food, approximate measure, and weight	Water %	Calories	Protein	Fat (Total lipid)	Saturated	Oleic	Linoleic	Carbohydrate	Calcium	Phosphorus	Iron	Vitamin A	Thiamine	Riboflavin	Niacin	Ascorbic acid
			gm	gm	gm	gm	gm	gm	mg	mg	mg	IU	mg	mg	mg	mg
Apricots:																
Raw, 3 med (107gm)	85	55	1	tr	—	—	—	14	18	25	.5	2,890	.03	.04	.6	11
Canned, in heavy syrup, 1 cup (halves and syrup) (258gm)	77	220	2	tr	—	—	—	57	28	39	.8	4,490	.05	.05	1.0	10
Avocados:																
Raw, 1 med (216gm)	74	370	5	37	5.5	22.0	3.7	13	22	91	1.3	630	.24	.43	3.5	30
Bananas:																
Raw, 1 med (119gm)	76	100	1	tr	—	—	—	26	10	31	.8	230	.06	.07	.8	12
Blackberries:																
Raw, 1 cup (144gm)	85	85	2	1	—	—	—	19	46	27	1.3	290	.04	.06	.6	30
Cantaloupe: ½ med (477gm)	91	80	2	tr	—	—	—	20	38	44	1.1	9,240	.11	.08	1.6	90
Cherries:																
Raw, sweet, 10 cherries (68gm)	80	45	1	tr	—	—	—	12	15	13	.3	70	.03	.04	.3	7
Cranberry juice: 1 cup (253gm)	83	165	tr	tr	—	—	—	42	13	8	.8	tr	.03	.03	.1	81
Fruit cocktail:																
Canned, 1 cup (255gm)	80	195	1	tr	—	—	—	50	23	31	1.0	360	.05	.03	1.0	5
Grapefruit, raw:																
Pink or red, ½ grapefruit (241gm)	89	50	1	tr	—	—	—	13	20	20	.5	540	.05	.02	.2	44
Sections, white, ½ grapefruit (241gm)	89	45	1	tr	—	—	—	12	19	19	.5	10	.05	.02	.2	44
Grapefruit juice:																
Fresh, 1 cup (246gm)	90	95	1	tr	—	—	—	23	22	37	.5	20	.10	.05	.5	93
Grapes, raw:																
Thompson seedless, 10 grapes (50gm)	81	35	tr	tr	—	—	—	9	6	10	.2	50	.03	.02	.2	2
Grape juice: 1 cup (253gm)	83	165	1	tr	—	—	—	42	28	30	.8	—	.10	.05	.5	tr
Lemon: 1 med (74gm)	90	20	1	tr	—	—	—	6	19	12	.4	10	.03	.01	.1	39
Lemonade: from frozen concentrate, 1 cup (248gm)	89	105	tr	tr	—	—	—	28	2	3	.1	10	.01	.02	.2	17
Orange: 1 med (131gm)	86	65	1	tr	—	—	—	16	54	26	.5	260	.13	.05	.5	66
Orange juice: from frozen concentrate, 1 cup (249gm)	87	120	2	tr	—	—	—	29	25	42	.2	540	.23	.03	.9	120
Peaches, raw:																
Whole, 1 med (100gm)	89	40	1	tr	—	—	—	10	9	19	.5	1,330	.02	.05	1.0	7
Sliced, 1 cup (170gm)	89	65	1	tr	—	—	—	16	15	32	.9	2,260	.03	.09	1.7	12
Pears:																
Raw, 1 med (164gm)	83	100	1	1	—	—	—	25	13	18	.5	30	.03	.07	.2	7
Pineapple:																
Raw, diced, 1 cup (155gm)	85	80	1	tr	—	—	—	21	26	12	.8	110	.14	.05	.3	26
Canned, heavy syrup, 1 cup (255gm)	80	190	1	tr	—	—	—	49	28	13	.8	130	.20	.05	.5	18
Plums:																
Raw, 1 plum (66gm)	87	30	tr	tr	—	—	—	8	8	12	.3	160	.02	.02	.3	4
Raisins:																
Dried, 1 sm pkg (14gm)	18	40	tr	tr	—	—	—	11	9	14	.5	tr	.02	.01	.1	tr
Raspberries, red:																
Raw, 1 cup (123gm)	84	70	1	1	—	—	—	17	27	27	1.1	160	.04	.11	1.1	31
Rhubarb:																
Cooked with sugar, 1 cup (270gm)	63	380	1	tr	—	—	—	97	211	41	1.6	220	.05	.14	.8	16
Strawberries:																
Raw, 1 cup (149gm)	90	55	1	1	—	—	—	13	31	31	1.5	90	.04	.10	.9	88
Tangerine: 1 med (86gm)	87	40	1	tr	—	—	—	10	34	15	.3	360	.05	.02	.1	27
Watermelon:																
1 wedge 4"x8" (926gm)	93	110	2	1	—	—	—	27	30	43	2.1	2,510	.13	.13	.9	30

tr = trace

Table of Nutritive Values of the Edible Part of Foods

(Dashes show that no basis could be found for computing a value although there was some reason to believe that a measurable amount of the constituent might be present.)

Food, approximate measure, and weight	Water %	Cal-ories	Pro-tein	Fat (Total lipid)	Fatty Acids Satu-rated	Unsaturated Oleic	Lino-leic	Car-bohy-drate	Cal-cium	Phos-pho-rus	Iron	Vitamin A	Thia-mine	Ribo-flavin	Nia-cin	Ascor-bic acid
			gm	gm	gm	gm	gm	gm	mg	mg	mg	IU	mg	mg	mg	mg
GRAIN PRODUCTS																
Breads, rolls, etc:																
Biscuit, baking powder 1 (2″ diam.) (28 gm)	27	105	2	5	1.2	2.0	1.2	13	34	49	.4	tr	.08	.08	.7	tr
Corn muffin, 1 muffin (40 gm)	33	125	3	4	1.2	1.6	.9	19	42	68	.7	120	.10	.10	.7	tr
White bread, enr, 1 slice (25 gm)	36	70	2	1	.2	.3	.3	13	21	24	.6	tr	.10	.06	.8	tr
Whole wheat bread, 1 slice (28 gm)	36	65	3	1	.1	.2	.2	14	24	71	.8	tr	.09	.03	.8	tr
Rye bread, light, 1 slice (25 gm)	36	60	2	tr	tr	tr	.1	13	19	37	.5	0	.07	.05	.7	0
Plain enriched roll, 1 med (28 gm)	31	85	2	2	.4	.6	.4	15	21	24	.5	tr	.11	.07	.9	tr
Hard roll, 1 med (50 gm)	25	155	5	2	.4	.6	.5	30	24	46	1.2	tr	.20	.12	1.7	tr
Danish pastry (4¼″ diam.) (65 gm)	22	275	5	15	4.7	6.1	3.2	30	33	71	1.2	200	.18	.19	1.7	tr
Cakes:																
Angel food, 1 piece (53 gm)	34	135	3	tr	—	—	—	32	50	63	.2	0	.03	.08	.3	0
Chocolate (chocolate frosting), 1 piece (1/16 of cake) (69 gm)	24	235	3	8	3.1	2.8	1.1	40	41	72	1.0	100	.07	.10	.6	tr
Fruitcake, dark, 1 slice (1/30 of loaf) (15 gm)	18	55	1	2	.5	1.1	.5	9	11	17	.4	20	.02	.02	.2	tr
Cupcake, plain, 1 (2½″ diam.) (25 gm)	26	90	1	3	.8	1.2	.7	14	40	59	.3	40	.05	.05	.4	tr
Pound cake, 1 slice (33 gm)	16	160	2	10	2.5	4.3	2.3	16	6	24	.5	80	.05	.06	.4	0
Doughnuts (cake type) 1 (2½″ diam.) (25 gm)	24	100	1	5	1.2	2.0	1.1	13	10	48	.4	20	.05	.05	.4	tr
Cookies:																
Vanilla wafers, 10 cookies (40 gm)	3	185	2	6	—	—	—	30	16	25	.6	50	.10	.09	.8	0
Sandwich type, 4 cookies (40 gm)	2	200	2	9	2.2	3.9	2.2	28	10	96	.7	0	.06	.10	.7	0
Brownies, 1 bar (20 gm)	11	85	1	4	.9	1.4	1.3	13	9	27	.4	20	.03	.02	.2	tr
Crackers:																
Graham, plain, 2 sq (14 gm)	6	55	1	1	.3	.5	.3	10	6	21	.5	0	.02	.08	.5	0
Saltine, 2″ sq, 4 (11 gm)	4	50	1	1	.3	.5	.4	8	2	10	.5	0	.05	.05	.4	0
Cereals (prepared):																
Bran flakes (40%) (fortified), 1 cup (35 gm)	3	105	4	1	—	—	—	28	19	125	12.4	1,650	.41	.49	4.1	12
Corn flakes (fortified), 1 cup (25 gm)	4	95	2	tr	—	—	—	21	(*)	9	.6	1,180	.29	.35	2.9	9
Puffed wheat, 1 cup (15 gm)	3	55	2	tr	—	—	—	12	4	48	.6	0	.08	.03	1.2	0
Shredded wheat, 1 biscuit (25 gm)	7	90	2	1	—	—	—	20	11	97	.9	0	.06	.03	1.1	0
Wheat flakes (fortified) 1 cup (30 gm)	4	105	3	tr	—	—	—	24	12	83	(*)	1,410	.35	.42	3.5	11
Cereals (cooked):																
Cream of wheat, 1 cup (245 gm)	89	105	3	tr	tr	tr	.1	22	147	113	(*)	0	.12	.07	1.0	0
Oatmeal, 1 cup (240 gm)	87	130	5	2	.4	.8	.9	23	22	137	1.4	0	.19	.05	.2	0
Cereal products:																
Macaroni, enr, cooked, 1 cup (140 gm)	73	155	5	1	—	—	—	32	11	70	1.3	0	.20	.11	1.5	0
Noodles, egg, cooked, 1 cup (160 gm)	71	200	7	2	—	—	—	37	16	94	1.4	110	.22	.13	1.9	0
Rice, white, enriched, cooked, 1 cup (205 gm)	73	225	4	tr	.1	.1	.1	50	21	57	1.8	0	.23	.02	2.1	0
Spaghetti, enr, cooked, 1 cup (140 gm)	73	155	5	1	—	—	—	32	11	70	1.3	0	.20	.11	1.5	0
PIES																
Apple, 1/7 cut (135 gm)	48	345	3	15	8.9	6.4	3.6	51	11	30	.9	40	.15	.11	1.3	2
Lemon meringue, 1/7 cut (100 gm)	47	305	4	12	3.7	4.8	2.3	45	17	59	1.0	200	.09	.12	.7	4
Mince, 1/7 cut (135 gm)	43	365	3	16	4.0	6.6	3.6	56	38	51	1.9	tr	.14	.12	1.4	1
Pumpkin, 1/7 cut (130 gm)	59	275	5	15	5.4	5.4	2.4	32	66	90	1.0	3,210	.11	.18	1.0	tr
FATS AND OILS																
Butter: 1 pat (5 gm)	16	35	tr	4	2.5	1.0	.1	tr	1	1	tr	150	tr	tr	tr	0
Margarine: 1 pat (5 gm)	16	35	tr	4	.7	1.9	1.1	tr	1	1	tr	170	tr	tr	tr	0
Cooking fats:																
Lard, 1 tbsp (13 gm)	0	115	0	13	5.1	5.3	1.3	0	0	0	0	0	0	0	0	0
Vegetable fats, 1 tbsp (13 gm)	0	110	0	13	3.2	5.7	3.1	0	0	0	0	—	0	0	0	0
Salad dressings:																
Commercial, mayonnaise type, I tbsp (15 gm)	41	65	tr	6	1.1	1.4	3.2	2	2	4	tr	30	tr	tr	tr	—
French, 1 tbsp (16 gm)	39	65	tr	6	1.1	1.3	3.2	3	2	2	.1	—	—	—	—	—
Mayonnaise, 1 tbsp (14 gm)	15	100	tr	11	2.0	2.4	5.6	tr	3	4	.1	40	tr	.01	tr	—

tr = trace

*varies with brand – see package label

APPENDIX B (CONTINUED)

Table of Nutritive Values of the Edible Part of Foods

(Dashes show that no basis could be found for computing a value although there was some reason to believe that a measurable amount of the constituent might be present.)

Food, approximate measure, and weight	Water %	Cal- ories	Pro- tein	Fat (Total lipid)	Fatty Acids Satu- rated	Fatty Acids Unsaturated Oleic	Fatty Acids Unsaturated Lino- leic	Car- bohy- drate	Cal- cium	Phos- pho- rus	Iron	Vitamin A	Thia- mine	Ribo- flavin	Nia- cin	Ascor- bic acid
			gm	gm	gm	gm	gm	gm	mg	mg	mg	IU	mg	mg	mg	mg
Salad or cooking oils:																
Corn, 1 tbsp (14 gm)	0	120	0	14	1.7	3.3	7.8	0	0	0	0	—	0	0	0	0
Soybean-cottonseed blend, hydrogenated, 1 tbsp (14 gm)	0	120	0	14	2.4	3.9	6.2	0	0	0	0	—	0	0	0	0
Olive, 1 tbsp (14 gm)	0	120	0	14	1.9	9.7	1.1	0	0	0	0	—	0	0	0	0
Safflower, 1 tbsp (14 gm)	0	120	0	14	1.3	1.6	10.0	0	0	0	0	—	0	0	0	0
Soybean, hydrogenated, 1 tbsp (14 gm)	0	120	0	14	2.0	5.8	4.7	0	0	0	0	—	0	0	0	0
SUGARS AND SWEETS																
Chocolate: plain, 1 oz (28 gm)	1	145	2	9	5.5	3.0	.3	16	65	65	.3	80	.02	.10	.1	tr
Honey: 1 tbsp (21 gm)	17	65	tr	0	0	0	0	17	1	1	.1	0	tr	.01	.1	tr
Jams and preserves: 1 tbsp (20 gm)	29	55	tr	tr	—	—	—	14	4	2	.2	tr	tr	.01	tr	tr
Syrup: table blend, 1 tbsp (21 gm)	24	60	0	0	0	0	0	15	9	3	.8	0	0	0	0	0
Sugar: 1 tbsp (12 gm)	1	45	0	0	0	0	0	12	0	0	tr	0	0	0	0	0
MISCELLANEOUS																
Beer: (3.6% alcohol) 12 oz (360 gm)	92	150	1	0	0	0	0	14	18	108	tr	—	.01	.11	2.2	—
Carbonated beverage: Cola type, 12 oz (369 gm)	90	145	0	0	0	0	0	37	—	—	—	0	0	0	0	0
Nuts: Peanuts, roasted, 1 cup (144 gm)	2	840	37	72	13.7	33.0	20.7	27	107	577	3.0	—	.46	.19	24.8	0
Peanut butter, 1 tbsp (16 gm)	2	95	4	8	1.5	3.7	2.3	3	9	61	.3	—	.02	.02	2.4	0
Pizza: (cheese), 1 (4¾″ pc) (60 gm)	45	145	6	4	1.7	1.5	0.6	22	86	89	1.1	230	.16	.18	1.6	4
Popcorn: plain, 1 cup (6 gm)	4	25	1	tr	tr	.1	.2	5	1	17	.2	—	—	.01	.1	0
Soups, canned: Beef noodle, 1 cup (240 gm)	93	65	4	3	.6	.7	.8	7	7	48	1.0	50	.05	.07	1.0	tr
Tomato, made with milk, 1 cup (250 gm)	84	175	7	7	3.4	1.7	1.0	23	168	155	.8	1,200	.10	.25	1.3	15

tr = trace

APPENDIX C

Estimated Safe and Adequate Daily Dietary Intakes of Additional Selected Vitamins and Minerals[a]

	Age (years)	Vitamins Vita- min K (µg)	Vitamins Biotin (µg)	Vitamins Panto- thenic Acid (mg)	Trace Elements[b] Copper (mg)	Trace Elements[b] Manga- nese (mg)	Trace Elements[b] Fluo- ride (mg)	Trace Elements[b] Chro- mium (mg)	Trace Elements[b] Sele- nium (mg)	Trace Elements[b] Molyb- denum (mg)	Electrolytes Sodium (mg)	Electrolytes Potassium (mg)	Electrolytes Chloride (mg)
Infants	0-0.5	12	35	2	0.5-0.7	0.5-0.7	0.1-0.5	0.01-0.04	0.01-0.04	0.03-0.06	115-350	350-925	275-700
	0.5-1	10-20	50	3	0.7-1.0	0.7-1.0	0.2-1.0	0.02-0.06	0.02-0.06	0.04-0.08	250-750	425-1275	400-1200
Children	1-3	15-30	65	3	1.0-1.5	1.0-1.5	0.5-1.5	0.02-0.08	0.02-0.08	0.05-0.1	325-975	550-1650	500-1500
and	4-6	20-40	85	3-4	1.5-2.0	1.5-2.0	1.0-2.5	0.03-0.12	0.03-0.12	0.06-0.15	450-1350	775-2325	700-2100
Adolescents	7-10	30-60	120	4-5	2.0-2.5	2.0-3.0	1.5-2.5	0.05-0.2	0.05-0.2	0.1-0.3	600-1800	1000-3000	925-2775
	11+	50-100	100-200	4-7	2.0-3.0	2.5-5.0	1.5-2.5	0.05-0.2	0.05-0.2	0.15-0.5	900-2700	1525-4575	1400-4200
Adults		70-140	100-200	4-7	2.0-3.0	2.5-5.0	1.5-4.0	0.05-0.2	0.05-0.2	0.15-0.5	1100-3300	1875-5625	1700-5100

a Because there is less information on which to base allowances, these figures are not given in the main table of the RDA and are provided here in the form of ranges or recommended intakes.

b Since the toxic levels for many trace elements may be only several times usual intakes, the upper levels for the trace elements given in this table should not be habitually exceeded.

Reproduced from: Recommended Dietary Allowances, ninth edition (1980, in press), with the permission of the National Academy of Sciences, Washington, DC.

APPENDIX D

Table of desirable weights for men and women aged 25 and over
(in pounds according to height and frame, in indoor clothing)

Height		Small frame	Medium frame	Large frame
Men				
Feet	Inches			
5	2	112-120	118-129	126-141
5	3	115-123	121-133	129-144
5	4	118-126	124-136	132-148
5	5	121-129	127-139	135-152
5	6	124-133	130-143	138-156
5	7	128-137	134-147	142-161
5	8	132-141	138-152	147-166
5	9	136-145	142-156	151-170
5	10	140-150	146-160	155-174
5	11	144-154	150-165	159-179
6	0	148-158	154-170	164-184
6	1	152-162	158-175	168-189
6	2	156-167	162-180	173-194
6	3	160-171	167-185	178-199
6	4	164-175	172-190	182-204
Women				
4	10	92- 98	96-107	104-119
4	11	94-101	98-110	106-122
5	0	96-104	101-113	109-125
5	1	99-107	104-116	112-128
5	2	102-110	107-119	115-131
5	3	105-113	110-122	118-134
5	4	108-116	113-126	121-138
5	5	111-119	116-130	125-142
5	6	114-123	120-135	129-146
5	7	118-127	124-139	133-150
5	8	122-131	128-143	137-154
5	9	126-135	132-147	141-158
5	10	130-140	136-151	145-163
5	11	134-144	140-155	149-168
6	0	138-148	144-159	153-173

Desirable weight tables are based on the concept that once growth in height has ceased there is no biological need to gain weight and that (as reflected by mortality and morbidity data) persons in their early 20's who are of average or less-than-average weight, have the best prognosis for good health. Desirable weight tables are applicable to persons aged 25 and older; measurements of weight and height are to be made with the subject in indoor clothing and shoes.

The Chart is adapted from insurance tables which are derived from the 1959 Build and Blood Pressure Study, Society of Actuaries. Three frame sizes are used, with a range of weights for each rather than a single weight. Unfortunately, no indication is given as to how to estimate frame size.

APPENDIX E

Approximate cholesterol content of selected foods*

Item, portion	Size	Cholesterol per edible portion
	gm	mg
Beef:		
Cooked, trimmed, 4 oz	113	102
Cooked, untrimmed, 4 oz	113	106
Brains: cooked, no fat added, 3 oz	85	2674
Butter: 1 pat	7	18
Cheese:		
Cheddar and processed, 1 oz	28	28
Cottage, creamed, 4% fat, 1 cup	245	48
Cream, 1 oz	28	32
Spreads and cheese foods, 1 oz	28	19
Chicken, turkey: cooked, 4 oz	113	102
Cream:		
Light (20% fat), 1 tbsp	15	11
Half and Half (12% fat), 1 tbsp	15	6
Egg:		
Whole, 1 med	50	252
White, 1 med	33	0
Yolk, 1 med	17	252
Fish:		
Lean and medium fat, cooked – haddock & halibut, 4 oz	113	70
Very fat, cooked – mackerel and herring, 4 oz	113	110
Gefilte fish: 3 oz	85	54
Heart: cooked (beef), 3 oz	85	233
Ham:		
Cooked, trimmed, 4 oz	113	99
Cooked, untrimmed, 4 oz	113	101
Ice cream:		
Rich, 16% fat, 1 scoop	71	40
Regular, 10% fat, 1 scoop	71	28
Ice milk: 1 scoop	71	14
Kidney: cooked, no fat added, 3 oz	85	683
Lamb:		
Cooked, trimmed, 4 oz	113	113
Cooked, untrimmed, 4 oz	113	113
Lard: (and other animal fat), 1 tbsp	14	14-17
Liver:		
Cooked, no fat added – beef, 3 oz	85	372
Chicken, 3 oz	85	634
Margarine: (all vegetable fat), 1 pat	7	0
Mayonnaise: (and mayonnaise-type salad dressing), 1 tbsp	14	8
Milk:		
Fluid, whole, 1 cup	244	34
Fluid, skim, 1 cup	246	5
Fluid, 1% fat, 1 cup	246	14
Pork:		
Cooked, trimmed, 4 oz	113	99
Cooked, untrimmed, 4 oz	113	101
Shellfish:		
Clams, 4 oz	113	71
Lobster, 4 oz	113	96
Shrimp, cooked, 4 oz	113	170
Crabs, 4 oz	113	113
Sweetbreads: cooked, 3 oz	85	396
Tongue:		
Cooked fresh, 3 oz	85	119
Cooked smoked, 3 oz	85	179
Veal:		
Cooked, trimmed, 4 oz	113	112
Cooked, untrimmed, 4 oz	113	114

Note: Cholesterol is not present in foods of plant origin such as fruits, vegetables, cereal grains, legumes, nuts, or oils.

*Feeley RM, Criner PE, Watts BK: *J Amer Dietetic Assoc 61*:134-149, 1972.

Obesity standards
for Caucasian Americans[1]
(minimum triceps skinfold thickness in millimeters indicating obesity)[2]

Age	Skinfold measurements	
(years)	Males	Females
5	12	14
6	12	15
7	13	16
8	14	17
9	15	18
10	16	20
11	17	21
12	18	22
13	18	23
14	17	23
15	16	24
16	15	25
17	14	26
18	15	27
19	15	27
20	16	28
21	17	28
22	18	28
23	18	28
24	19	28
25	20	29
26	20	29
27	21	29
28	22	29
29	23	29
30-50	23	30

1. Adapted from Seltzer CC, Mayer J: A simple criterion of obesity. *Postgrad Med 38*: 101-107, 1965.

2. Figures represent the logarithmic means of the frequency distributions plus one standard deviation.

Mean heights and weights and
recommended energy intake

Category	Age (years)	Weight (kg)	Weight (lb)	Height (cm)	Height (in)	Energy needs (with range) (kcal)	(MJ)
Infants	0.0-0.5	6	13	60	24	kg x 115 (95-145)	kg x .48
	0.5-1.0	9	20	71	28	kg x 105 (80-135)	kg x .44
Children	1-3	13	29	90	35	1300 (900-1800)	5.5
	4-6	20	44	112	44	1700 (1300-2300)	7.1
	7-10	28	62	132	52	2400 (1650-3300)	10.1
Males	11-14	45	99	157	62	2700 (2000-3700)	11.3
	15-18	66	145	176	69	2800 (2100-3900)	11.8
	19-22	70	154	177	70	2900 (2500-3300)	12.2
	23-50	70	154	178	70	2700 (2300-3100)	11.3
	51-75	70	154	178	70	2400 (2000-2800)	10.1
	76+	70	154	178	70	2050 (1650-2450)	8.6
Females	11-14	46	101	157	62	2200 (1500-3000)	9.2
	15-18	55	120	163	64	2100 (1200-3000)	8.8
	19-22	55	120	163	64	2100 (1700-2500)	8.8
	23-50	55	120	163	64	2000 (1600-2400)	8.4
	51-75	55	120	163	64	1800 (1400-2200)	7.6
	76+	55	120	163	64	1600 (1200-2000)	6.7
Pregnancy						+ 300	
Lactation						+ 500	

The data in this table have been assembled from the observed median heights and weights of children shown in Table 1,* together with desirable weights for adults given in Table 2 for the mean heights of men (70 inches) and women (64 inches) between the ages of 18 and 34 years as surveyed in the U.S. population (HEW/NCHS data).

The energy allowances for the young adults are for men and women doing light work. The allowances for the two older age groups represent mean energy needs over these age spans, allowing for a 2% decrease in basal (resting) metabolic rate per decade and a reduction in activity of 200 kcal/day for men and women between 51 and 75 years, 500 kcal for men over 75 years and 400 kcal for women over 75 (see text). The customary range of daily energy output is shown for adults in parentheses, and is based on a variation in energy needs of ± 400 kcal at any one age (see text and Garrow, 1978), emphasizing the wide range of energy intakes appropriate for any group of people.

Energy allowances for children through age 18 are based on median energy intakes of children these ages followed in longitudinal growth studies. The values in parentheses are 10th and 90th percentiles of energy intake, to indicate the range of energy consumption among children of these ages.

*"Table 1," "Table 2," and "text" in this legend refer to material in the book Recommended Dietary Allowances.

Reproduced from: Recommended Dietary Allowances, ninth edition (1980, in press), with the permission of the National Academy of Sciences, Washington, DC.

SUGGESTED READING

Schneider HA, Anderson C, Coursin D (eds): Nutritional Support of Medical Practice. New York, Harper & Row, 1977.

Chaney MS, Ross ML, Witschi JC: Nutrition, ed 9. Boston, Houghton Mifflin, 1979.

Davidson S, Passmore R, Truswell AS, Brock JS: Human Nutrition and Dietetics, ed 7. New York, Churchill Livingstone, 1979.

Deutsch RM: Realities in Nutrition. Palo Alto, Bull Publishing, 1976.

Nutrition Misinformation and Food Faddism, Nutrition Reviews, Special Supplement, July 1974, Nutrition Foundation.

Present Knowledge in Nutrition, ed 4. Nutrition Foundation, 1976.

Stare FJ, McWilliams M: Living Nutrition, ed 2. New York, John Wiley & Sons, 1977.

Thorn GW, Adams RD, Braunwald E, Isselbacker KJ, Petersdorf RG (eds): Harrison's Principles of Internal Medicine, ed 8, part 4, section 1. New York, McGraw-Hill, 1977.

Whelan EM, Stare FJ: Eat OK – Feel OK. N. Quincy, Mass, Christopher Press, 1978.

ACKNOWLEDGMENTS

David B. Coursin, MD   Figure 46

John H. Crandon, MD   Figure 55

William J. Darby, MD   Figure 49

M. Edward Davis, MD   Figure 60

Thomas R. Dawber, MD   Figure 1A

James M. Dunning, DDS   Figure 32

Bernard S. Epstein, MD   Figures 23, 27, 58

Stanley N. Gershoff, PhD   Figure 45

M. K. Horwitt, PhD   Figures 38, 39

Norman Jolliffe, MD   Figure 20

Robert F. Littlefield, Jr   Figure 4

Richard H. Lyons, MD   Figure 44

F. J. Margolis, MD   Figures 5, 6, 8, 9

Karl E. Mason, PhD   Figure 59

Rustin McIntosh, MD   Figure 54

Metropolitan Life Insurance Company   Appendix D

C. V. Moore, MD   Figure 52

Hildery A. Nelson, MD   Figures 24, 26

Rosa Lee Nemir, MD   Figures 56, 57, 58

Blair C. Rich, DDS, FICD   Figures 7, 31, 33

Karl Singer, MD   Figure 48

Charley Smith, MD   Figure 53

Alfred Sommer, MD   Figures 16, 17, 18

Tom Spies, MD   Figures 36, 37, 43

INDEX

References to illustrative material are in boldface type